BEDTIME STORIES FOR ADULTS

COGNITIVE BEHAVIORAL THERAPY FOR INSOMNIA

Relaxing lullabies and daily exercises based on cbt techniques to help you fall asleep. Overcome stress, anxiety and depression

Kirsten Wallace

Table of Contents

Introduction 1

Chapter 1. About CBT.. 9

Chapter 2. A Tropical Island 19

Chapter 3. Edward the Conqueror 31

Chapter 4. Flying Tigers...................................... 43

Chapter 5. The Old Menu (24 min)..................... 55

Chapter 6. The Hot Air Balloon Ride 65

Chapter 7. The Wandering Tribe 77

Chapter 8. Planter's Life 85

Chapter 9. Home Sweet Home 95

Chapter 10. The Sleeping Beauty in the Wood 105

Chapter 11. Autumn Dreams 115

Chapter 12. Forsaken Among The Forsaken........ 127

Chapter 13. A Fishy Tale 137

Chapter 14. Mozart Moon 149

Chapter 15. The Sleep Blossoms 157

Chapter 16. The Lovebirds 167

Chapter 17. Floating Forever Downstream.......... 177

Chapter 18. Honolulu Dreams........................ 185

Chapter 19. Lisa Bakes A Cake 193

Chapter 20. The Black Ball 205
Chapter 21. The Right Choice 215
Chapter 22. The Pokémon Monster.................... 225
Chapter 23. New Orleans 237
Chapter 24. The Bell of Atri 243
Chapter 25. The Mermaid................................ 251
Chapter 26. Finding Shorty 263
Chapter 27. A Trip Into Starlight...................... 273
Chapter 28. The Award-Winning Story 287
Chapter 29. Quiet Night In The Forest 297
Chapter 30. Count Neighbors........................... 309
Chapter 31. Animal Dreams 319
Chapter 32. Taking Flight In Dreamland............ 333
Chapter 33. Water For The Queen 347
Chapter 34. The Old Woman 357
Chapter 35. Dandelion Wish 365
Chapter 36. Beneath The Waves 377
Chapter 37. All I Have Got 387
Chapter 38. The Rookie Detective 397
Chapter 39. Wet Dreams................................. 407
Chapter 40. Spanish Trip 415
Chapter 41. The Writer 421
Chapter 42. Mark 431

Chapter 43. The Dimensional Life Coach 443

Chapter 44. The Stairway Between Realms 453

Chapter 45. Lemonade 459

Chapter 46. Lost City in the Woods 467

Chapter 47. Grape Harvest.............................. 477

Chapter 48. Ambien 487

Conclusion... 497

Introduction

First, let's talk about why do bedtime stories matter?

Mindfulness, relaxation, and hypnotizing the body into a pleasant sleep is a key part of all this. The stories that you heard were whimsical tales, and while they might have seemed like much as a child, when looking back on this as an adult, it played a major role in our lives.

Bedtime stories were fun to hear. Sometimes, your parent would do voices. Other times, they'd just read the books quietly, and you'd pay attention each time. Sometimes they'd be tales you've heard plenty of times, other times they were tales they fabricated on a whim.

Do you remember some of your former bedtime stories?

If you do, do you remember how they made you feel? The words you heard? The imagery you'd remember?

All of this plays a key role in why bedtime stories for adults are so important, and why, with each story you hear, you feel relaxed, at ease, and of course, able to sleep.

Each story will have fun, whimsical ideas, or imagery of different scenarios that you've been through before. The quests that you have, and even, a sleep fairy that will help you sleep. With every single story, you'll be spirited away on a wonderful adventure, one that's fun for you, and a good trip for everyone in the story.

If you have trouble falling asleep, just imagine yourself in the different scenarios each of these wonderful characters go through. As you get spirited away in this adventure, you'll notice that, with each time, and each place, it'll change for you. There are many different aspects to consider with each story, and many adventures to be had.

Also, don't think you'll hear the same story twice. While it might be the same words, there might be new adventures to be had, and new ideas that come forth.

Bedtime stories for adults also help with taking your attention off the troubles of life. Whether it be work, bills, or even your family that stress adds up and it can make it hard for you to fall asleep. Many adults suffer from insomnia or can only sleep for a certain period of hours. That combined with the incredibly long work weeks, and also with the early morning shifts, it's not easy out there. But, with these bedtime stories, you'll relax your mind, you'll take your attention off the troubles you have, and promote relaxation, and of course sleep with each word you hear.

Many adults benefit from these types of stories. Some of us might wonder why, but if you take a moment to think about it, when was the last time you weren't focused on the stresses at hand, but instead on a relaxing, fun bedtime story that will help with sleep. If you can't remember, then you need these bedtime stories for adults.

With each story, each word uttered, each sound you hear, I hope they will lull you to sleep. It helps as well with shutting off your brain, helping you get focused on the different words you hear, and instead of feeling stressed and depressed, you'll get your mind off the troubles you have, and instead, feel brighter than ever.

So, sit back, get comfortable, and listen to these relaxing bedtime stories. And with every one of these, you'll feel yourself whisked away into the tales they tell, and hopefully, you'll have pleasant dreams and a wonderful sleep as you continue to hear each story, and the creative, relaxing, and inspiring tales each one of them has to offer.

Passive Thought Observation

We would park our bicycles at the base of the hill and walk halfway up this gently rolling hill. It would be not too bright nor too gloomy. It was just right. Sure enough, the clouds would roll by, and my friends would have so much fun just describing what the clouds looked like.

The funny thing is that one friend would say a certain cloud looked like an elephant, and another friend would say that it looked like a Volkswagen.

Clouds can look like whatever you want them to look like, and your answer is no better than the person sitting next to you. You're constantly reading your personal meaning on to cloud shapes. You acknowledge the clouds and they move on.

What if I told you that you can adopt the same attitude with your thoughts? This is called Passive Thought Observation. It's a mindfulness practice where you close your eyes and follow your breathing patterns and focus on your thoughts.

However, instead of normal thought processes where you try to grab a hold of your thoughts and judge them and connect them with other things, you consciously do something else. Instead of getting emotionally worked up by your thoughts, choose to just look at your thoughts as they flash in and out of existence in your mind. This activity is similar to being a little kid again, reclining against that hill with your arms folded looking at the clouds. You think one cloud looks like one thing only for the cloud to be replaced by another which looks like something else completely different.

Passive Thought Observation is a very powerful mindfulness practice because it enables you to free yourself and the automatic emotional connection you have with your thoughts. You know you no longer feel like you have to judge. There is no need for you to feel that you have to always be in control. Instead, you give yourself permission to let things go.

Ironically enough, when you do this you actually take greater control of your thought processes.

Anybody can adopt Passive Thought Observation. It has a few simple stages; first, you need to count your breath; second, you need to achieve an internal state of peace; third, you have to train your mind's eye to the thoughts forming in your head. Finally, you train yourself to withhold judgment. Just acknowledge the thoughts. No need to analyze or over think things different.

Passive Thought Observation is a very powerful mindfulness practice because it enables you to free yourself and the automatic emotional connection you have with your thoughts. You know you no longer feel like you have to judge. There is no need for you to feel that you have to always be in control. Instead, you give yourself permission to let things go. Ironically enough, when you do this you actually take greater control of your thought processes.

Anybody can adopt Passive Thought Observation. It has a few simple stages; first, you need to count your breath; second, you need to achieve an internal state of peace; third, you have to train your mind's eye to the thoughts forming in your head. Finally, you train yourself to withhold judgment. Just acknowledge the thoughts. No need to analyze or over think things

Chapter 1. About CBT

Cognitive Behavioral Therapy or CBT is a well-known evidence-based treatment used for anxiety and depression. It's been around for almost five decades now so there's a huge chance that you've already heard about it. Aside from the conditions mentioned, CBT is also used for the treatment of chronic pain, as well as a host of other emotional and mental ailments.

Beck is considered the father of cognitive behavioral therapy, as well as of cognitive therapy. He pioneered a number of theories that are now being used in the treatment of various anxiety disorders, as well as of clinical depression. It was Beck who developed the self-report measures of depression and anxiety, one of which is the Beck Depression Inventory or BDI, which is now one of the most widely used tool for measuring the severity of depression among patients.

Beck first came up with his theory on CBT in the late 60's. Many saw it as a parry to the psychodynamic and Freudian approaches to mental health that became very influential during that era, both of which focused on unraveling a patient's past and placing the patient under long-term therapy. Beck's approach was different. He focused instead on the thoughts of the individual and the notion that how a person thinks affects how he feels. If a person can control his thoughts and change them, he can have control over his emotions and change them at will.

In other words, cognitive behavioral therapy is a short-term therapy approach that can help individuals discover new ways you respond to certain situations by changing the way they think. What separates CBT from traditional approaches that are psychodynamic, and insight- and past-oriented is that its focus is the present. It asks the following questions:

"What are you currently thinking about?"

"What were the things you were thinking of before you felt the anxiety?"

"What do you do whenever you start feeling angry?"

Obviously, the goal of this approach is to understand what's going on in your brain and body when your emotions begin to overwhelm you. And unlike traditional approaches, the source is not something that happened in your past but what is happening in your brain at the moment.

How Does CBT work?

The main focus of cognitive behavioral therapy is on the relationship between a person's thoughts, feelings, and behaviors. CBT operates on the fundamental concept that events in themselves do not and cannot provide emotional turmoil. On the other hand, it's the person's perception of things and the meanings they assign to events that cause it. Therefore, if a person can change their relationship with preconceptions or troubled memories, then they can change their perception.

In CBT, what the therapist does is take an engaging approach to pinpointing unhealthy thought patterns, deeply rooted principles and beliefs, and behavioral patterns. The moment these elements are identified, the therapist begins working with the patient, helping them replace unhealthy coping mechanisms with more appropriate, healthier solutions.

An individual's thoughts and feelings play a major role in their behavior. For instance, someone who spends a lot of time thinking about car crashes and road accidents may find themselves always feeling unusually nervous when commuting.

The goal of CBT is to train patients into thinking that while they may not be always in control of every aspect of the world they live in, they can take control of the way they interpret things and the way they deal with their environment.

During a CBT therapy session, the therapist may ask you regarding your past, particularly your childhood. This is for the therapist to have a better understanding of the kind of environment you grew up in, such as whether there may be a history of mental health problems in your family. The focus then is on understanding what's going on inside of you every time emotional problems arise.

In other words, therapy is about increasing your self-awareness, helping you understand why you think the way you think, why you react a certain way when you're stressed or anxious, or even when you're depressed or in pain.

What things does your mind focus on? What does your self-talk look like? What do you say to yourself whenever you're feeling down and can't seem to get out of bed in the morning? What do you do when someone says something that offends you? For CBT, awareness is the first step to change. It's only when a person becomes aware of their reactions that they can begin to change them. This includes both thoughts and behaviors. It's important to note, though, that the change CBT brings about is not immediate. Even if you are able to change your thought patterns, you can still expect your feelings to stay the same for some time.

You will still feel guilty for saying no to an invitation to be part of the PTA at the school your child is attending. You will still feel anxious that you were not able to get all your chores done on time. And you are still likely to feel depressed if you try to force yourself out of bed.

The reason for this is that emotions lag behind your thoughts and behaviors. It will take several repetitions of creating new thoughts and behaviors for your feelings to finally get in sync.

Every habit you have is represented by a formation of circuits in your brain, and no, they are not easy to reconstruct. At the same time, it's also important to reward yourself for every milestone you achieve breaking unhealthy thought and behavioral patterns.

The theoretical roots of CBT can be traced back as early as 1913, during the beginnings of behaviorism as pioneered by John B. Watson whose work laid the foundation for a lot of CBT's concepts. After that, it was also heavily influenced by the work of Albert Ellis on Rational Emotive Behavioral Therapy (REBT) in the 1950s as well.

With that said though, it's actually Dr. Aaron T. Beck that most consider to be the formal founder and first pioneer of Cognitive Behavioral Therapy (CBT).

Instead, what he observed was that most of his clients often had internal experiences (thoughts and feelings) that significantly impacted their behaviors and led them to develop a lot of the psychological distress and mental health problems for which they sought professional help for. This "internal dialogue", as he called it, impacted their perceptions and attitudes towards a certain person or situation in ways many of them did not realize. "This is so hard. The therapy isn't working and I'll never get better," and thus, start to become more resistant, despondent, and apathetic towards both the therapist and their condition.

Because of this, Beck started to conceptualize depression in terms of the streams of impulsive, negative thoughts that his depressed patients often struggled (and failed) to overcome. He coined the term "automatic thoughts" to refer to this phenomenon and posited that people interact with the world through their mental representations of it (i.e., thoughts, ideas, and belief systems). Thus, if a person's mental representation or reasoning is inaccurate or dysfunctional, then their feelings and behaviors may become problematic.

He investigated the kinds of automatic thoughts that seemed to be most common among his clients and categorized them as: negative ideas about the self; negative beliefs about the world; and negative views of the future.

With this, he got to work on how to identify and correct these automatic thoughts. This emphasis on thought processes was the reason why Beck initially labeled his approach as simply "Cognitive Therapy" instead of "Cognitive-Behavioral Therapy."

He helped his patients identify their own automatic thoughts and encouraged them to think more objectively and consider things more realistically. Once they corrected their underlying beliefs, it became easier for clients to stop their maladaptive behaviors and conquer their feelings of depression, anxiety, guilt, trauma, and negativity. This would eventually lead them to emotional relief and allowed them to function better as a whole.

With that said, however, CBT as a field of study has gone beyond the work of Aaron Beck and has now become an umbrella term for many different therapeutic techniques with the same fundamental elements and assumptions.

One example of this is Albert Ellis' Rational Emotive Behavior Therapy (REBT), which we mentioned earlier. Similar to Beck's CBT, REBT is a kind of cognitive therapy that seeks to resolve a client's emotional and behavioral issues through correcting their irrational beliefs. It was from Ellis' work that much of Beck's ideas originated.

Dr. Judith Beck, the daughter of Aaron Beck, is another important proponent of CBT as she did a lot to continue her father's work through her research and development of better CBT techniques. She also encouraged positive coping mechanisms in her clients. Now she is widely regarded as the foremost expert authority on CBT and one of the best and most skilled CBT therapists working today.

Currently, CBT is the most empirically validated and effective form of psychosocial intervention in the world of clinical practice. It has gone on to inspire more than a thousand research papers and has been used to treat a number of mental health problems and psychological disorders. Aside from that, CBT also owes a great deal of its popularity to its success in treating many of society's most prevalent mental disorders, such as eating disorders, anxiety disorders, mood disorders, trauma-related disorders, and more.

With that said, the field has certainly come a long way since it began over half a century ago, and it remains relevant and beneficial to this day. Many experts would agree that Cognitive-Behavioral Therapy (CBT) has undoubtedly become an integral cornerstone not just in clinical psychology and therapy, but in self-help and mental wellness as a whole.

Chapter 2. A Tropical Island

"Can eel firm wife da dolphins 'gain, Mommy?"

"Finish brushing your teeth first!" Jenny called into the bathroom.

The silly child poked her head out of the bathroom, toothbrush in hand, lips covered in toothpaste.

"Okie, Mom!" Flecks of toothpaste flew as she said it, and then grinned with foamy teeth.

Kirsty came out wiping her mouth with the back of her long sleeve and hopped into the bed as Jenny pulled back the covers.

"I really like the dolphins, Mom. They know how to have fun!"

"They do." Jenny nodded. "But there are all kinds of dreams to explore, you know. There is an entire world full of them out there. All kinds of perspectives you never imagined."

"What does 'perspective' mean, Mommy?"

Jenny tapped a finger to her lips. "It's...it's a way you view the world. Do you know how you got to see the forest dreaming from the fox's view? That's a new perspective."

"Oh, okay! So what kind of per-spec-tie are we going to see tonight?"

Jenny opened the book, it is cover crackling.

"Oh, yes. This is a special one."

She turned the book so that Kirsty could properly see the picture.

It depicted a tropical island, thick with palm trees and ferns, and fallen coconuts on the beach forming a pattern that looked like the numeral "3."

Above it, in the swaying branches and green canopy, peeked all sorts of brightly colored birds.

Their many calls mingled with the sound of the lapping waves to create a light and hopeful background.

The scent of salt and the pungent fragrance of tropical plants drifted from the pages.

"Now, sweetie, let me show you what the dolphins were so keen to get to explore, but from a different perspective...."

Jaina woke up on a beach, but not the beach she had left.

Now instead of a sandy path back to the city, she found herself on a tropical island.

Coconuts littered the sand at her feet.

Bright red and spiky fruits hung in some of the trees.

A warm tropical wind blew past, stirring the leaves with a whispering rustle and billowing her hair. Jaina smiled as she breathed it in. The air smelled so fresh, a lingering tang on her tongue. She turned toward the nearby jungle. A small bird with green feathers and a shiny blue around its head hopped down from one of the branches. "Welcome!" it chirped. "This is my home. Do you like it?" Jaina nodded enthusiastically. "It's wonderful. So warm and cozy and peaceful. How do you ever stay awake here? I think I would spend my day napping if I lived in such a nice place!"

"Oh, but you don't know what else there is to see!" said Bird. "You would have no time for napping all day if you could see the beauty of this place!"

"Could I? Could you show me?" Jaina looked hopeful, her eyes big and bright. A bird could not resist her plea. "Yes, I will show you. Come with me and see what only one on the wing can see! Then you tell me if you would spend all day napping."

"Deal!"

Jaina held out her arm, and Bird alighted upon it, tilting its head back and forth to stare at her with each eye. "And...let the wind takes us!"

Then it flew off again, and Jaina found that she was looking at the beach from high above.

She was like Bird, winging her way through warm blue skies to appreciate the jungle and the ocean from on high. She circled higher and higher, and the whole island became a green-carpeted seed below her. Up until this high in the sky, only the winds kept her company, singing of the distant waves, of the past and the future.

"Here we go!" Bird dove down, tucking her wings, as the green jungle rushed up to meet her. She spread her wings and arced smoothly into level flight, circling the treetops.

Below her, she saw the coconuts sitting in the trees, humming softly in the breeze.

Harsh voices rose up to meet her: monkeys leaping from branch to branch, picking the fruits and eating them with lyrical delight.

They looked up at Bird as she flew past and waved their hands in envy. Into the canopy, she plunged. Green fan-shaped leaves fluttered in the wind as she flew past. Other birds, some of them yellow with black beaks, and some of the dark blue with yellow beaks, and still others red with white markings sang loudly, all competing voices. They looked up as she flew past. Some rose into the air with a flutter of feathers, but they could not keep up with her speed.

She wove through corridors of green and tan, leaves and branches adorned with fruits or coconuts, nimbly winging around tree trunks, dodging hanging vines, and great big spider webs glistening with morning dew like living chandeliers.

The chorus of chirps and hooting cries followed her as she raced through a blur of the jungle. Then she was free and flew out over the beach, above the water. Fish leaped and swam in the cerulean waves, all aglow from the sunshine warming the world. Dolphins cavorted off the shore, leaping high from white-capped waves to glisten in the sun and crash back down again. Bird Jaina watched the shadows darting about beneath the surface, and then she turned back to the island. Flocks of seabirds circled on the shores, diving down to peck at some meal washed ashore. "Food! Food! Food!" their cries said. The bird had more on her mind than simply eating.

She circled the island, white sand streaming by beneath her, the lush jungle rotating slowly in her eyes. Slender fingers of sunlight crept through the canopy and golden dust swirled in their grasp.

Little lizards and dark beetles crawled up the trunks, racing to the top to reach the sunlight. Their voices rose ever higher in competition. The bird let out a warbling song to drown them out. Her voice echoed in the jungle as she spiraled ever higher, eventually reaching high above the island once more. "This is an amazing view!" said Jaina.

"Yes, it is." Bird tucked her wings and dove once more. "But sometimes you need to see from a bird's eye view up close!" Down she flew into the jungle canopy, landing upon a high branch.

The wind caressed her feathers as she preened her wing, and then looked down on the world unfolding below her. In the thick undergrowth, many creatures crawled, each with a voice of its own.

A furry anteater hummed its slow, ponderous song as it wandered lazily through the brush, long tongue flicking out of its long face. The anteater stopped and looked up at Bird as she sang down to it. "Good...morning..." said the anteater, it is every word drawn out and rolling.

"It is a good morning!" said Bird. "But there are no ants up here, my friend."

"That's...okay." The anteater plodded along on its search.

A soft croak drew her attention, followed by another, and another. Small frogs with very vibrant coloring hopped up the tree trunk. Bird knew better than to test them: they were beautiful but dangerous if you were careless, much like the sweetest of dreams. One of the frogs, neon green with red sides, leaped from the tree as a wind sighed through the palm fronds.

The frog spread into wings of luminous glass, a butterfly with glowing blue and black patterns on its wings.

As Bird and Jaina watched the butterfly shattered into a hundred tiny slivers of blue light, and each grew wings, a sudden swarm of sky-blue butterflies shining in the shaded forest canopy.

Laughing, Bird flew down to join them, and suddenly found herself caught within a cloud of swirling blue. They spiraled with the wind, down nearly to the ground and then back up into the branches, pushing through the leaves and emerging into the sunlight beyond.

As the butterflies flew, a symphony of fluttering notes filled the air. The bird stopped flapping her wings and for a moment just drifted up on the music of the island itself: the rush of wings, wind, and waves, all joining together to create a warm sound.

The frond-leaves were as wings, emerald feathers joining her in flight. Whole flocks rose out of the green to take to the sky with her, and they soared so high even the wind envied them. Blue skies opened up before them, and to Jaina's delight, she found they soared higher still. Into kingdoms of cloud they flew, where mountains of mist and moisture rolled past, and visions of the ancient world rose up and fell away in mere moments.

Clouds became like islands in the sky, floating upside down in an airy ocean.

The wind rolled through it all like oceanic currents, some warm and lazy, some cool and swift.

The flock changed again, leaves borne upon the wind, now clad in white cloud-feathers, wreathed in a scent of rain. Thunder rolled and the islands gave way to a downpour, cascading from the clouds as waterfalls. The flock dove into the rain, becoming like fish of sea green, fins like wings, but the music never changed. The song of the island: that of sea and sky, where the voices of the waves and the dreams of the wind combined.

Therefore, down they fell, back into the water, bursting through the surface and emerging from a geyser of bubbles in yet another world. There the deep blue embraced them, warm and salty, and they sank into its liquid softness. Currents enveloped them.

Colorful ocean fish darted back and forth amid the reefs that surrounded the island, and the flock changed yet again, becoming like them, bright and quick, yet trailing seaweed from their tails. Longer and longer, the trails grew, as they flew through the water around the island, binding it in green.

Exercise

Mind the Mouth

TIME TO READ: 3 MINUTES

TIME TO DO: 7 MINUTES

Mindful eating is an easy way to practice your new skills—after all, you'll have at least three opportunities each day. There's no single way to eat mindfully. This exercise is about being aware of what you are eating and focusing on enjoying the moment. Eliminate other distractions, such as scrolling through social media, watching TV, or finishing homework. Rather, take a moment to look at, think about, smell, and savor your food.

1. Take three deep breaths. Place your food on your plate or in your bowl and look at it.
2. While taking three more deep breaths, think about the source of your food—the fields, farms, or ocean it came from.
3. Take three more deep breaths while thinking about the delicious smell.
4. Take three more deep breaths. Take a bite and notice the temperature, flavor, and texture of the food. As you chew, notice the sensations

and the release of flavors in your mouth. As you swallow your food, note the sensations and the remaining flavors in your mouth.
5. After you finish the first bite, place your utensils down and take three deep breaths. Repeat the exercise until you are full.
6. Finish by taking three deep breaths.

Chapter 3. Edward the Conqueror

Louisa grasped a dressing material, ventured out of the entryway of the kitchen behind the house into the chilly October daylight. She was sitting tight for the man who might before long fix the lift.

"Edward, she called! It's prepared for lunch!"

A second, she quit, tuning in, and afterward went to the grass, a little cloud went over her, and strolled over a seat, tenderly brushing the sundial with one hand as she moved by.

She was reasonably pleasant about a young lady who was little and stout, a slight lilt in her direction, and a delicate development of her hands and her legs.

"Lunch Time!" She was now able to see him, maybe at this time he was about a seventy feet away, down in the plunge on the base of the woods the kind of tall, thin man in khaki pants and dim pullover that was green, remaining adjacent to a significant blaze with a fork in his mouth, hurling thistles on to the highest point of the fire. It was thundering energetically, billows of white smoke emanating from the orange flames below. The smoke was floating over the nursery with a beautiful aroma of fall and consuming leaves. Maria went down the incline towards her dad. In the event that she wished, she may likely have made another call before she opened her eyes and allowed herself to see, however, there was something in particular about a five-star campfire that prompted her to move towards it, straight very nearby, such that she was able to feel the warmth and hear it out consume.

"Lunch," she stated, drawing closer.

"Oh, hi. Okay —yes. I'm going."

"What a decent fire."

"I've chosen to gather this spot straight up," her dad said.

"I'm wary of every one of these briers."

His gloomy look was clammy with sweat. There are little drops of it staying on his mustache like dew, and two small streams were trickling down his neck on to the turtleneck of the pullover.

"You should be cautious; you don't try too hard, Edward."

"Maria, I do wish you'd quit tending to me just as I was eighty."

"No doubt, truly, I get it. A tad of activity never hurt anyone." God, Henry! Edward! Edward! Gracious! Look! Look! Goodness! Look! Look!" The fellow turned and took a gander at Maria now, who indicated the furthest side of the fire. "That pooch! The cat!" It was a fabulous enormous feline on the planet lying close to the light, so flares frequently observed him hitting him, so he held discreetly, with his face in the sky from one viewpoint and his ears, and keeping a quiet yellow eye on his man and woman." Maria shouted, at that point she immediately dropped the treat, got it with both her arms, whisked it away, and set it on the blazes free grass.

"Your insane cat," she said, tidying off her feet.

"The spouse let me know," Cats recognize what they are doing. You won't discover a feline doing whatever they don't care for.

"Whose is it? Not felines."

"Ever before you saw it?"

"Actually, I haven't."

The feline was perched on the grass, and taking a gander at it parallel, with an inside, hidden articulation, something inquisitively omniscient and thinking and a fragile demeanor of scorn around the nose, as though seeing these two individuals, the one little, full, and ruddy, the other sweeper and sweet, was somewhat solemn.

"Be an average cat now and go on home to where you have a spot."

Her man, a significant other, started pacing around the slanted road that led to the house. The pussy cat got up and sought after, away off first, anyway edging ever closer as they came. After a short time, it was near to them; by that time, it was well in front of everyone else, similarly pacing as it asserted the entire spot, with its tail held straight open to address, like a post.

"Come all the way back," said the man. "Go on home. We needn't bother with you."

Nevertheless, at the moment when they hot home, it followed them inside, and Maria served it some warm milk inside a bowl. As everyone was enjoying their lunchtime meal, it ricocheted up to the additional seat and persevered though the lunch session with its head busy gazing at what is on the dining table.

"I couldn't care less for this cat," protested Edward.

"Goodness, I trust it's a fine catlike. I do believe it stays a brief span." Directly, listen to me, Maria. The creature can't in any capacity whatsoever stay here. It has a spot with someone else. It's lost. Moreover, if it's up 'til now endeavoring to remain close by tonight, you should take it to the police. They'll see it comes all the way back."

Immediately after Edward was don taking his lunch, he returned to his development. Maria, as anyone may have guessed, went straight to the piano. She was an experienced piano player and a real music sweetheart, and every other night, she always dedicated an hour or two of her time just to play on her own. By now, the cat was lying comfortably on the lounge chair, and as she controlled stroking it as she cruised by, the cat simply opened its eyes, looked around briefly before resuming its nap.

"You're a terribly not too bad catlike," she said. "Besides, such dazzling concealing. I wish I could keep you."

Her fingers then gently slid on top of the stairway and onto the cat's head and came across a little lump, a slight bump right over the cat's right eye.

"I feel pity for his cat," she said. "You have thumped on your first face. You ought to get old."

She walked over to the piano, sat on the long piano stool, but she was not so quick to start playing. One of her one of a kind little delights was to make a customary kind of show day, with an intentionally composed program that she figured out the detail before commencing. She was not mainly a fan of breaking pleasure by stopping while she considered what to play straightaway. All that she required was a short relief after every piece, as she was very busy gathering of onlookers hailed energetically and needed extra. It was such a lot of increasingly lovely to imagine a horde of individuals, and sometimes as she was busy playing, she was able to see an unending stockpile of chairs and what seemed to be a sea made up of white faces improved in her direction, tuning in with a bolted and admiring core interest. Occasionally, she enjoyed playing a tune or two from her memory, and sometimes she would play a song that she had overheard somewhere; that was the manner by which she felt. Moreover, what should the program be? She took a seat in front of the keyboard with her little palms got on her legs, a heavy reddening minimal individual with an around and still lovely face, she had done her hair up in an ideal bun that formed at the top of her head.

By gazing imperceptibly on to the other side, she was able to see that the cat had already settled comfortably into the love seat, and I was just amazed by the way that its dull fur lay flawlessly against the purple color of the cushion.

Shouldn't something be said about some Bach in any case? Or then again, far, and away superior, Vivaldi.

An uncommonly respectable program, one that she possessed the ability to adequately play it without the music. She edged herself nearer the piano and postponed every other time whenever a person from the group - starting at now she was able to feel like this was one of her lucky days; at the time, a person from the gathering of onlookers had just had his final hack; by then, with the moderate ease that went with about the total of her advancements, she anchored her hands up against the support and started playing.

At that specific moment, she was not paying much attention to the cat, and was also unable to view the cat in any way shape or form - to be sure she had disregarded its quality - yet as the significant primary notes of the Vivaldi carefully filled the room with a melodious sound, and from the corner of a single eye, of an unexpected hurricane, a blast of improvement on the love seat on her correct side. She quit playing pronto.

"What is it?" she asked as she went to get her cat. "What's going on?"

The animal, who two or three minutes before had been resting tranquility, was directly sitting straight up on the couch, it was tense with the whole-body quivering, the ears were pointing straight up, and its eyes during the entire distance remained open, and all the time its gaze was fixated on the piano

"Did I alarm you?" she carefully asked.

"You have probably never listened to some good music before."

"No," she said, I just do not feel like it is what it is. On apprehensions, she couldn't resist touching that the cat like's mien was not one of fear. There was no contracting or venturing back. In the event that anything, there was a slanting frontward, a type of fervor regarding the animal, and the face- - well, there was to some degree an odd attitude on the front, something of a mix among stun and paralyzed.

Clearly, the substance of a cat is a slight and straight forward thing, anyway if you are observant enough to notice how the eyes and ears coordinate circumspectly, and for the most part that small area of flexible skin underneath the ears and hardly to the opposite side, you can at times watch the impression of inconceivable sentiments. Maria was watching the face eagerly now, and in light of the fact that she was quite intrigued to witness what will happen in the ensuing time, she associated her hands to the reassurance and started playing the Vivaldi.

Exercise

Emotions in Motion

TIME TO READ: 3 MINUTES

TIME TO DO: 7 MINUTES

Emotions come from our mood, circumstances, and relationships with others. We label these feelings as good or bad. One technique for managing emotions is to acknowledge them and shift them in the opposite direction. Research has shown that smiling—even when we feel down—can help our body produce serotonin and dopamine, the happy hormones.

No matter how you feel emotionally, use this exercise to shift your feelings because—this is important to remember—emotions are about how you feel about something and you can easily control them using exercises like this one. This exercise will use 2 + 4 breathing.

1. Close your eyes and take a moment to note your emotions.
2. While doing 2 + 4 breathing, notice where in your body the emotion is located and place your hands over that area.

3. Smile and say to yourself or out loud, "I choose happiness." Repeat the phrase.
4. While doing 2 + 4 breathing again, smile and open your eyes. Notice the shift in your emotions. Repeat the phrase 10 times.

Chapter 4. Flying Tigers

The older adult heard a far off thundering and turned his eyes to the sky. He was seeking a gravely required downpour to guarantee a full collection. "A cloudless sky," he murmured. Out there, he thought he saw a herd of dark flying creatures flying in an exceptional example. At that point, he saw men running rapidly from the fields yelling, "It is the Japanese!" The ranchers would be the fortunate ones today. The individuals who lived in the city were most certainly not.

The Japanese aviators took an enjoyment watching individuals on the ground dispersing like mice. They snickered and yelled "Banzai" to one another. Executing was such a simple errand against such an unprotected populace.

Before long there would be no resistance to Japan's requirement for painfully required assets. The Emperor required nourishment for his kin, work for his industry, and oil to keep up Japan's military mastery.

The Far East would turn out to be a piece of his Empire. The Chinese, they guaranteed, ought to be thankful for their new sovereign ... all things considered, they were "freeing" the Chinese from the "remote fallen angels."

Their celebration was hindered by the shouting sound of planes originating from above. The rear turret heavy armament specialist's eyes enlarged in dread at seeing a warplane with the substance of a fearsome tiger shark painted on its nose.

"Flying Tigers!" the kids yelled, while the grown-ups pulled them to security. When resistance to those "noxious dwarves" from Japan appeared to be vain, it was seeing these bold American pilots that were viewed as a blessing from their divine beings. Each time one of the aircrafts was taken out of the sky in a wad of fire or seen diving to the earth, there was an extraordinary cheering from the workers.

One of the pilots accompanying one of the Mitsubishi Ki-21 "Sally" overwhelming aircraft, named "Sally's" by the Americans, got maddened by his powerlessness to get the escaping tigers and looked for retaliation by strafing a gathering of youngsters who had walked out reasoning that the threat had passed. They could see the pilot chuckling as the slugs tore through the little one's bodies sending them flying into the air like cloth dolls.

"That son of bitch!" yelled Ricky Caruso, one of the "Tigers" who had seen the slaughter. He put his nose into a lofty jump and started to pound the Ki-27 with slugs from his .50-gauge nose weapons. The pilot zigged and zoomed Caruso's P-40 War hawk's unrivaled speed yet in a plunge found the "Nate," and inside seconds, the plane was ablaze. He could see the Japanese pilot squirming miserably as the blazes devoured his substance.

'Consume in Hell, you charlatan!' Ricky's idea as he pulled up from his plunge.

"Post Rico!" a yell came over the radio. "You have a Jap on your tail!" Ricky went to look when he saw slugs tear into his conservative. He dunked his wing and went into a shallow jump wanting to evade his assailant.

"Try not to attempt to battle him, Rico! That little dark-colored jerk's unreasonably agile for you. I'm coming, simply keep him off of your tail."

Ricky zigged and crossed; however, the Japanese pilot was resolved to get his retribution. 'I figure I may have gotten it this time,' he thought. He felt a crash hit the rear of his seat secured by a thick defensive layer plate and realized that the following slug might discover him.

Out of nowhere, he heard one of the Tigers plunging and saw tracer projectiles flying past him. He saw the Jap contender, another Nakajima Ki-43, or "Oscar" as the Americans alluded to it, fly away with a severely harmed tail fold. There was yelling over the radio, and things like: "Go get that jerk," and "make him meet his progenitors," yet the Tiger let him go and reacted in an unmistakable and quiet Midwestern drawl: "I'll get him next time."

Ricky perceived the voice. It was his best and dearest companion, Lars "Bull" Lundgren, the stumbling ranch kid from Minnesota. He heard the thunder of a motor to one side and saw Ox's whole toothed smile gazing back at him.

"I owe you one!" Ricky snickered, yet the trial had obviously shaken him.

Volunteers

The one thing you learn in the military is never to chip in, or so the platitude goes, yet the children of the Great Depression knew whenever there was a chance to be had, you needed to bounce on it. Ricky and Ox were two of those children.

Ricky and Ox were the two most improbable companions that one could envision. Ricky was a wiry minimal Italian-American child from New Jersey with a smart mouth and a belligerent disposition. The bull was a rancher's child from America's heartland... a blundering monster of Swedish stock, calm, with a quiet aura that gave a false representation of his high astuteness. The two of them made them thing in like manner. They were acceptable with anything mechanical and wanted to fly.

There was a genuine push by the American Government to reinforce its air corps. During the middle of the Depression, Hollywood turned out movies that celebrated pilots as legends, confronting peril in the skies. They longed for turning out to be Aces, that is, to score at any rate five executes against the adversary. Why stop at five. Most likely, the Red

Baron's score of eighty must be outperformed? Wasn't America the best nation on the planet?

The war in China had been continuing for very nearly ten years when they get for Volunteers turned out in March of 1941. The Russians had been helping the Chinese battle the Japanese, yet now was pulling out and making a beeline to meet the more noteworthy risk from Hitler. The German war machine was traveling through Poland and smashing the entirety of the Soviet protections.

Chiang Kai-Shek, the pioneer of the Nationalists in China, approached the American Government, on edge that Japan's authority in Asia would go unchecked, for help. Ricky and Ox thought nothing about China, yet they realized that a war was approaching between Imperial Japan and the United States.

"We got to get right now they come here!" was the catchphrase heard everywhere throughout the airbases the nation over. The pilots were all the while flying the old biplanes and were kicking the bucket to get their hands on the new Curtiss P-40's.

Ricky and Ox met in flight school. They alternated being the tops in their group, however, Ricky pushed out Ox in the aeronautical battle moves and didn't let him overlook it.

"Hello, Ox!" Ricky cried. "Com'ere, take a gander at this."

Bull, who was never one to be excessively energized, gradually strolled over to his companion who was on his toes attempting to peruse the note that some insightful ass nailed high to the release board.

"Put me down, douche bag!" Ricky reprimanded as he wriggled out of the large man's hold.

"I didn't see a stepping stool 'round here so I figured you might require a lift" Ox giggled.

"Tune in up Ox. It says here that they need fliers in China. Volunteers will be released from the equipped administrations, to be utilized for "preparing and guidance" by a private military contractual worker, the Central Aircraft Manufacturing Company (CAMCO). They'll pay $600 every month for pilot officials, $675 per month for flight pioneers, $750 for squadron pioneers and about $250 for talented ground crew

49

members. A portion of the folks said that they would get 500 bucks for each Jap that they destroy!"

"I don't know, and you need to leave the Army to join. Is it accurate to say that you are certain you need to change it for an undertaking?"

"Listen to Ox. On the off chance that we get over yonder and kill a few Japs and become Aces, at that point we could bring in some decent cash, return with fight understanding, and re-enroll. We can't lose... except if... you're a major chicken?"

"They call me Ox, not chicken. Alright, little man, I'm in!"

That mid-year, Ox, Ricky, and around 100 other "volunteers"' boarded ships bound for Burma conveying regular citizen visas. They were at first based at a British runway in Tango for preparing while their airplane was amassed and test flown by CAMCO staff at Mingaladon Airport, only outside of Rangoon. General Chennault, the establishing pioneer of the American Volunteer Group, set up a school building that was made fundamental because numerous pilots had "lied about their flying experience, guaranteeing interest experience when they had flown just aircraft and once in a while considerably less ground-breaking planes.

It wasn't some time before each man had his image spankings' new P-40 War hawks that the Brits turned down as out of date. They would confront the Japanese warrior, the Nakajima Ki-27, a slower, yet progressively agile contender in the hands of an accomplished flier. Chennault cautioned them not to be maneuvered into a dogfight. On the off chance that they had to draw in, the men were advised to place their plane into a lofty jump and pull up quickly. Any Japanese pilot sufficiently silly to attempt to get them would separate in mid-air as they couldn't deal with the "G" powers in their delicate manufactured airplane.

Aircraft were focused on. P-40 pilots were told to swoop down like winged animals of prey from high heights and lay into the plane squadrons with overpowering firepower. "Hit them rigid," and get the damnation out of there!

"Presently it's close to home!"

Ricky and Ox were working off a headache when the news came:

"Hello Guys, get your butts out of bed! Fitz shouted. The Colonel needs everyone out as soon as possible. We got great news from Pearl Harbor!"

"I feel like poo!" Ricky groaned.

"You look like poo!" Ox giggled.

"You'll be in poop on the off chance that you don't get your rear ends up brisk" cautioned Fitz.

There was protesting among the youngsters as they bobbled on that early December morning. They sat in the field house hanging tight for the Colonel.

Exercise

Calm Breaths

TIME TO READ: 3 MINUTES

TIME TO DO: 7 MINUTES

Do you have a potentially stressful situation coming up? Maybe you have a big history test, or you had a fight with a friend and are worried about seeing them in school. Don't worry—this exercise will help you gain confidence and calm with mindful breathing.

1. In a quiet room, sit comfortably in a chair with your feet placed firmly on the ground. Gently rest your hands on your stomach. Set a timer for 7 minutes; use your phone if you don't have a timer handy.

2. Close your eyes and focus on your breathing. Breathe slowly until you can move the breath down to your belly. Place your hands on your stomach and feel it gently rise and fall.

3. While doing the 4, 7, 8 breathing (Yoga Breath), say to yourself or out loud, "I can confidently take care of my day." Repeat three times.

4. Return to breathing normally, with eyes closed, until the timer completes.

Chapter 5. The Old Menu (24 min)

Jack grabbed a jacket and an umbrella from his closet. He had thought of driving, but the rain wasn't coming down that hard. He was going to meet an old friend, in their favorite diner. He had not seen Carlos in close to a year.

The pair were inseparable as children. He could still remember the night they met. The fair was in town, and the smell of fried foods permeated the air around Jack. He was only ten, but he was already beginning to find his rebellious spirit. He wanted to ride all the "upside-down" attractions. His parents refused his requests, but he had worn them down enough to allow him to ride The Whisk.

The Whisk was a large metal abomination that jerked its passengers around, from one side to another. The seats allowed for two riders in each cab, but Jack was in a new town and he knew no one, so he sat alone. The ride appeared to be starting, but Jack could not fasten his seatbelt.

The ride operator was walking around with another young man. Jack did not hear the man saying anything, because he was on the other side of the attraction. He had apparently asked if anyone would be willing to take another passenger in their cab, as the boy was the odd number in his group.

Jack had enthusiastically raised his hand, in an effort to summon the operator's attention. The man thought that he was volunteering to take the extra boy, with an embarrassing enthusiasm. Thus, Carlos was seated next to Jack and the two began a life-long friendship. A friendship that just happened to begin with Carlos thinking that Jack was insane. Jack laughed to himself at the memory, trying not to cringe. His luck had always been a little weird. He opened the door from his building to the outside world. The rain had picked up quite a bit. He opened the umbrella and decided to take his chances anyway. Jack walked along the sidewalk, listening to the rhythmic tapping of the raindrops against the slippery fabric that protected him from the elements. He accidentally bumped into another pedestrian, apologizing profusely.

The restaurant was a tiny hole-in-the-wall sort of establishment. He and Carlos would eat lunch there almost every day when they were in college. The meatball hoagie was the stuff of miracles; he had never found a better tasting sub. Jack turned the corner to see that familiar aged brick exterior. There was a neon sign hanging in one window that said only "Hal's". He wondered for a moment, what sort of person Hal was. How had he never met Hal?

He opened the door to the diner, shaking off his umbrella outside before surrendering himself to the warmth of the building. Jack brushed his against the matt that lay in front of the threshold. A man behind the long wooden bar acknowledged him as sat down in a booth by the wall. Jack had missed this place. It smelled like grease and old wood, which doesn't sound nearly as pleasant as the scent actually was. He imaged that the atmosphere had not changed since the moment the diner was conceived and that he what he loved about the establishment.

There were tin photos of old actors and branded ads, adorning the wood-paneled walls. An old bulletin board in the corner held pictures of every regular. Hal's even had the classic framed dollar, supposedly the first to be exchanged at the restaurant.

There were only two lights in the dining area, and they were both hanging from the ceiling, attached to fans. This meant that the overall atmosphere was dimly lit and antiquated. He pulled the laminated menu from behind a metal napkin holder, flipping it over to find the hoagie.

To Jack's surprise, the menu had changed. Nothing looked the same. They seemed to have the basic fare, like burgers and hotdogs. There were no more subs and no hoagies.

The young man was not the sort to get worked up over trivial things, but he felt an aching in his heart. He had been remembering his past all day, with a heavy soul. Jack had let his friendship with Carlos drift away from him when his friend had moved. The missing hoagie was just enough to remind him how much had changed about his life.

Jack took a deep breath to calm his hurting spirit. He was not going to allow himself to be taken over by a single moment, especially not when he was about to see his friend. He used the other patrons in the diner to distract himself. At the table to the front of his own, sat a mother and her young son. He could only see a portion of the child's head, but he was immediately reminded of his youth. He had to stop remembering for just a few moments!

Jack watched an old man walking through the door with a smile upon his weathered face. He waved to the man behind the bar and took a seat in front of him. He could hear the men laughing to one another. Jack had become so engrossed in their conversation that he had neglected to watch the door. Carlos placed his hand upon Jack's shoulder. Jack hadn't seen him in so long, he could have wept. He stood up and embraced his old friend, whose jacket smelled of wet leather.

A waitress approached the table as Carlos found his seat. They both ordered a soda, Jack suspected that was because that's what they had always done. He looked his friend over. Time was such a strange beast. They were both still young, but so much had changed about their lives and their faces. Carlos looked tired, with pronounced shadows beneath his eyes. He had always been handsome but in an unusual way. His face was wide, and his cheeks were full. Jack had missed the glasses! He had almost forgotten about those thick-rimmed glasses. Carlos placed both hands upon the table and looked enthusiastically at his oldest friend.

"It has been too long. How have you been? You must tell me everything," said Carlos.

"I will, of course. What about you, though? How is your practice? Your wife?" Jack asked.

"I actually wanted to talk to you about that! There is something that I must tell you," Carlos said. He took his drink from the waitress. They told her that they would need a few moments before ordered and then they patiently waited for her to return to her place behind the bar.

"Tell me," said Jack.

"So, do you remember all those days in college? We would get lunch here almost every day," he said. Carlos ran his finger along with the chipped vinyl that covered the old tables. One of those tables should still carry an autograph from each of them.

"I do remember. I was just thinking about those days and how cruel time is. I miss having friends. I miss seeing you and all the dumb jokes that we would tell," said Jack.

"Well, miss no longer! I am returning to the city with Tracy. We are going to build our lives here. You and I will share so many new stupid memories and this is the last time that you will ever be nice to me. Don't think I don't remember who you really are," said Carlos, laughing. Jack felt his heart drop. New memories? This was the best news that he had heard in a long time. He had been lamenting his glory days so much, lately. He had completely forgotten that it was possible to make new memories.

"What? That is amazing! That is perfect!" Exclaimed Jack.

"Weird how this place never changes, huh? I think I may get the meatball hoagie, just for old-time's sake."

Exercise

Soundscapes

TIME TO READ: 2 MINUTES

TIME TO DO: 8 MINUTES

This exercise will teach you how to focus your attention, how to harness it, and how to maintain it. Humans have an amazing capacity for focus, but that doesn't mean it comes naturally. That's why we need to train our attention to stay where we want it to for as long as we need it.

In this exercise, you are going to focus on one simple thing: sound. What do you hear around you? If you focus, you'll probably find that different sounds are going on all around you: indoor sounds, outdoor sounds, even the sounds inside your own body, like heartbeats and breaths and your stomach growling. In this activity, we are going to learn how to keep our attention focused on those sounds and not let it wander.

1. Sit comfortably in a chair with your feet placed firmly on the ground, or sit on the floor with your legs in Half Lotus (crisscrossed legs) position. Rest your

hands on your knees or in your lap. Set your timer for 8 minutes.

2. Begin by focusing your attention on the sound of your breath flowing in and out. Start noticing other sounds around you. Let the various sounds arise, then be replaced by the next sound you notice.

3. Continue focusing only on sound. When your attention wanders, notice this, too, and gently bring it back to sound. Continue the exercise until your timer completes.

Chapter 6. The Hot Air Balloon Ride

Sometimes, all you need is to feel far from all of your cares and worries.

Sometimes, all you need is to glide through life on a serene cloud, floating across a pale blue sky.

If you have ever been on an airplane ride and looked out the window, then you have probably noticed the ethereal world above the clouds.

It is so calm and relaxing, high off the ground, and far away from all of the stress of life.

Have you ever taken a ride in a hot air balloon?

Have you ever been lifted off the ground slowly, like you were being carried by a gentle giant to a restful place?

Your journey into peacefulness and relaxation will begin on the ground, preparing for your journey of slow and tender flight, as you crawl slowly through the clouds in a comfortable basket.

Begin your ascent first by lying down in a comfortable position.

If your body needs to be adjusted at all to help you for the most comfort in this space, make those adjustments now before you enter a place of total stillness.

You are going to be carried away on the air, firstly through your breath.

Your breath will align you with your inner harmony and balance.

Your breath will help fill you with the peacefulness you desire and help you release all of the cares and worries you may be carrying around with you right now.

Every inhale is a beautiful source [of comfort, refreshment, and light.

Every exhale is a letting go, a release of tension, a movement closer to restful relaxation.

Breathe here for a few moments.

Connect to your body.

Connect to your feelings.

Connect to the sense of relief from your breath...

You are here to feel free from the world of deadlines and agendas.

You are here to only exist within yourself and your deeper sense of true peace and balance.

This practice of connecting to your physical body through your breath, and your spiritual essence through your creative mind, is what will help you to refresh your life-force energy and feel fully healed, refreshed and connected to your inner soul.

Your only purpose now is just to float through a heavenly landscape.

Underneath your body, you begin to feel the softness of grass on a majestic hillside.

It is a bright and beautiful, sunny day.

As you look up into the sky, you can see that it is full of the most glorious, puffy, white clouds.

You look over now and see the basket just walking distance away—the basket that will carry you far off into the heavens.

You are eager to go over to it and witness the gigantic balloon rise up off the ground, full of the hot air that will lift you up.

The basket is easy for you to climb into a much larger than you would have thought.

There is enough room inside for you to lie down in any direction.

The balloon is airing up while you are climbing inside.

It is starting to lift off of the grassy earth and align with the basket, to float over and hover above it.

You can feel yourself feeling elated but calm—excited, but relaxed.

Your path is up and up and up, and there is no other landscape, but the clouds on high.

You will get there soon.

Your balloon is almost ready to lift you up and all you have to do when the time comes is pull on the cord to send you off the ground.

Inhale deeply, slowly pulling fresh air into your lungs...and exhale gently out.

Again, inhale slowly and steadily, gathering all of the hot air you will need to soar high up in the clouds...and exhale.

Breathe out all of the cares and worries that will weigh you down.

Breathe away all of the tension that will keep your balloon on the ground...

You are ready, and your balloon is ready.

It's time to pull the cord and feel your ascent.

The cord is easy to pull.

It feels effortless as you give it a tug and release hot air into the giant balloon above your head.

The river is full of life, and it flows smoothly, cutting across the land as far as the eye can see, the sunlight of the day glistening on its surface.

The river becomes smaller and smaller as you float higher and higher, taking a deep breath in and exhaling gently...

You look to the west, and you see a great, wide forest that pushes far across the land.

The higher you go, the smaller the trees become, the wood of the branches and trunks disappearing behind the green foliage.

The tops of the trees, which once seemed so close, are now at a great distance from your hot air balloon.

You can feel the journey getting steadily closer to the clouds...

You look out of the basket to the south, and you see fields and meadows reaching far across the land, sewing a patchwork quilt of land as far as your eye can see to the south.

The lands of the farmers, the cattle, the goats and the sheep—the land of food that grows, of harvests and abundance from the fertile soil.

This land will stretch out for miles more, as your balloon gets ever higher, and can see that much farther across the land.

You look out to the north and are much higher now.

You begin to see the curve of the Earth from this height and feel completely restful as you look to the North Star, already visible from this height in the sky.

You have ascended to the atmosphere of the cloud world, and it is here that you will find your greatest peacefulness and comfort.

It is here that you can let all of your worries and cares drift off and away from you, falling back to the earth as you drift through the clouds...

Look around you as you inhale deeply and exhale smoothly.

You are completely surrounded by puffs of white moisture.

They look like giant cotton balls piled together in beautiful mounds of softness.

Your basket is moving slowly, but you feel the momentum of your balloon as it wafts on the breeze of the high atmosphere.

You have no trouble breathing here.

You can take deep, fulfilling breaths.

You can feel totally relaxed as you inhale and exhale from this point in the sky...

Breathe now as you let in the magnificent scenery of an all-white horizon fill your soul.

Breathe into this place of total calm and serenity.

Let the clouds high above the earth; comfort you.

You are warm here.

You are safe.

You have enough oxygen to breathe.

All you have to do is take in the majesty of this place.

The whole world above the clouds looks like a tundra of snow and ice for thousands of miles.

It looks angelic and full of bright light, the light from the sun reflecting off of the cloud faces.

Beneath the clouds is the whole landscape of the world you know—the world where you eat, sleep, work, love...

Let it come fully into your thoughts.

As you let it take shape in your thoughts, turn it into something you can hold in your hand, a physical object that represents this worry or stress...

It could be a heavy bag of sand that represents the weight that you feel from your work or your home life.

It could be a dollhouse to symbolize how you feel about your home or your living space.

It could be a person that has been upsetting you or weighing you down. Anything is possible from this place within your mind.

Do not judge yourself for how it comes up or how it forms.

Simply allow it to take shape so that you can hold it in your hands...

Notice the clouds again and the atmosphere you are floating again.

Reminding yourself of your stress may have brought up those feelings for you again.

Look out to the clouds.

You are here in a hot air balloon, free to just release the pain you are suffering, free to align with your highest consciousness and internal vibration of light...

Here you are, high above the clouds, facing your current anxiety or worry.

You are holding it in your hands, and you are ready to let it go.

You can hold it over the side of the balloon and prepare to let it go.

You are not hurting it, whatever it is.

It is a symbolic release of what has been holding you back from your relaxation and relief.

It is a symbolic action to cut the cords with your tension, worry, and doubt...

Hold the symbolic object over the edge and promise to let go of everything right here, right now.

You have no reason to hold onto this part of your life anymore.

You have no reason to doubt yourself.

You have no reason to fear to let go of this issue or these fears.

It is time.

Here, high above the clouds, it is time for you to say farewell to this part of your life.

It serves no purpose.

It only causes distress and discomfort.

Let it go.

Let it fall far away, through the clouds to wherever it must go.

Resolve to know that you are free of it.

Release it fully and take a nice, long breath in through your nose.

Hold your breath here for a moment, like you were holding the object over the side of the basket...and release the breath, letting it flow away from you.

Notice the serene landscape around you, unfolding as far as your eye can see...

You are safe here.

You are free.

You have released your discomfort.

You can now relax a little more and let yourself delve more deeply into your unconscious thoughts and dreams.

Here in the heavens, high above the soft, cotton-like clouds, you can prepare for your ascent farther and deeper into dreamland.

You will not return to the Earth tonight.

Tonight, you will continue to float high above the ground in your hot air balloon and find all of the relief you have been looking for.

Exercise

Monkey Moment

TIME TO READ: 2 MINUTES

TIME TO DO: 8 MINUTES

This exercise is a great technique for managing anxiety. Try imagining the anxiety inside you as a cute little monkey that worries about being left behind. Perhaps you could engage the monkey and have some compassion for its fears. Understand that you are much wiser than the monkey, so you can listen to its concerns and also choose how you feel about them.

1. Go to a favorite trail, a peaceful area, or simply take a walk in your neighborhood before you go to school. Set your timer for 8 minutes. Begin by walking slowly, placing one foot in front of the other—heel to toe.

2. While walking, repeat the positive self-mantra "May my monkey have peace."

3. As you say this, imagine the monkey calming down and resting on your back.

Chapter 7. The Wandering Tribe

This is the tale of the Wander Tribe. Long ago, there was a great empire that rested on the shores of a sea. The capital of the empire was a great metropolis that had been built over the course of countless centuries. No one truly knew how long it had been or for how long it would last. But there was a select few that feared. The fear was an unsteady breath in their lungs. It was a doubt in the back of their minds. A voice that kept whispering to them. It spoke so far away in a voice they could not understand. But that didn't stop the ones who heard the voice from gathering and proclaiming what was coming.

The Emperor didn't like this. In fact, he despised it. Who were these nay-sayers and doubters to sow the seeds of fear among his people? Prophets? There was no such thing. The Emperor did not trust in spirits and magic. He believed in science, engineering, and history. The hard studies of life that had guided him in his expansion of the empire. And so, he declared that these men and women, these fearmongers, were banished from their lands. They had one day to gather their things, pay their dues, say their goodbyes, and leave. If he found any within the borders of the capital after midnight, he'd burn them out.

It was a harsh and bitter fate for those who were only trying to protect their loved ones. They wanted to defend the empire that they called home. But to the iron-willed ignorance that the Emperor wielded, these men and women were powerless. So, without course to follow, they did as this man commanded. The so-called "Prophets and Fearmongers" gathered their meager belongings and traveled out into the hills beyond the capital. And just as midnight rolled over the horizon, doom came. As the voice protected, the empire burned. They choked on their greed. They bathed in their malice. They drowned under the weight of the chains they cast on those below. Inequity was nails in their coffins. The city literally erupted into an unearthly fire of green and purple light that burned long after they turned away from their failure.

The outcasts and sole survivors of this now fallen empire wandered for many decades. Generations were born of these few. Children that would never know the origins of their existence. The people did not know of another land that could care for them. There were no kingdoms or empires near this side of the earth that could give them a respite from their journey. They were sent out on a forced exodus. The journey went on for decades more. The generation born to wandering gave life to another generation. And so did the generation after them. Eventually, the band of exiles became a band of refugees. Then the band of refugees became a group of soul-survivors. And then the gathering of soul-survivors expanded into a tribe. The Wandering Tribe, they called themselves.

The history of who they were and where they had come from had drowned in the confusion of oral tradition. Their language twisted and transformed into something entirely new. Their written texts were few and far in between. Though there was land aplenty to wander, the leaders had trouble finding one that they should settle on. There was a small group of wanderers called the First Men and First Women. These were the leaders. Their ancestors were the first men and women to hear the Voice. Nobody knew who the Voice was or where it was, but it was always with them. It gave the First Men and First Women guidance. Through the insight of the Voice, they were protected and nurtured. Though they were without a home, they were given a plentiful number. Though they did not have much land, they accumulated a rich culture and range of skills. They prospered, despite the severe adversity they faced.

For many years from then, the First Men and First Women lead their people on through the endless journey. They theorized that lands might be infinite on earth, but the Voice must be somewhere upon it. Steadily, as they had traveled, the Voice's connection to them had become stronger. It was guiding them to land that it rested upon. And from what the First Men and First Women knew of their people's history, the whole reason they left the Lost Empire was because of the Voice. If they decided to settle down or give up now, all of this would have been for nothing.

But it was not! Eventually, after the years burned and expanses crossed, they discovered the land they had searched for. After so long, after such pain, the people of the Wander Tribe had discovered their savior and deliverer. For the longest time, they believed the Voice was a god of some kind. What they discovered was mildly disappointing. In the center of a snowy tundra, set high up in the mountains, there stood an obelisk of white stone. And upon that obelisk, flickering in the endless snows, was a silver-blue flame. The flame never vanished or wavered. It didn't die out in the cold and it had no source for fuel. For the longest time, the First Men and First Women wondered over what had created this magical light.

And then the Voice spoke up from it. This flame, this light, the magical substance, was the source of the Voice. Their god. Their guardian and guide over a century and a half of wandering. Some of the people were disappointed. They expected something awesome and all-powerful. Others looked for something more humanoid and relatable. But the First Men and First Women felt great peace in this flame's presence. So, they named it the Sacred Flame and declared that this would be their new home. They dismantled their carriages and used the wood to build homes. They hunted the woods and gathered furs. With patience and determination, they developed a new way of life in this alien land.

Centuries later, this Wandering Tribe would give life to the Chief Howlite of the First Men and Chieftess Lilith of the First Women. Under the guidance of the

Voice of the Sacred Flame, they grew powerful beyond belief. Beings of unimaginable power and mystical origin, the Chief and Chieftess ushered in a new era on the earth. During their supernatural lifespan, they rose their village into a city. From there, they transformed their city into a kingdom. Their kingdom rose into an empire. And their empire became an entire country. The Sacred Fire led them with many lessons that granted profound wisdom. The greatest lesson it ever taught Howl and Lilith was the lesson of the cycle. Life repeated itself; history turned like a wheel. What came before would come again. And by saving the people of the Wandering Tribe from extinction through a burning empire, it rebuilt a greater empire that reshaped the world.

Exercise

Connection Junction

TIME TO READ: 3 MINUTES

TIME TO DO: 7 MINUTES

Sometimes it's difficult to connect deeply with our emotions. The exercises in this book—like this one—were created to help you do just that. It is completely normal to feel overwhelmed by emotions. This exercise is about developing a way to sit calmly with all your emotions and not become consumed by them.

1. Find a comfortable position to meditate and set a timer for 7 minutes.

2. Begin by doing a round of 2 + 4 breathing. Slowly begin to notice your emotions, even if you can't identify them at first. Note where you feel them in your body. It could be tension in your back, or throbbing or lightness in your forehead, stomach, or chest.

3. When you note a sensation in your body, take a moment and say, "I feel . . ." and name the emotion.

4. Each time you say out loud, "I feel . . .," try to name the sensation in your body. Allow yourself to feel the feeling while releasing any negative aspects of the emotion.

5. End by repeating a round of 2 + 4 breathing. Repeat the entire exercise four more times.

Chapter 8. Planter's Life

Paul watered the daisies and tulips the same way he had for the past twenty years. For the last five, he did it alone.

Before then, he and Sheila spent their days together out in the sun in their paradise of a retirement home. Everything had come together exactly as they had hoped: the sunlight hit the soil at the exact angle they needed, and they chose a region that didn't get so hot as to boil the plants' water.

The two of them had the most extravagant garden in miles. Nothing nearby even came close. It took both of their hard work to get the garden to the state it was in, and after Sheila passed on, Paul was still thankful for what she put into their life's project.

An onlooker might see Paul and think of him as a simple gardener who toiled away in his remote country home for food. He didn't care one way or the other what people thought of him, but Paul knew himself to be more complicated and nuanced than your stereotypical farmer.

He knew there was a world outside the land he owned — he figured he had to be aware of it, for the way he saw it, he didn't have much land, to begin with.

They might have said it was a small dream to keep a flower and vegetable garden, but he knew that people who said such things didn't know how much work it was.

Taking care of plants was no small feat. Paul had to make sure each of them were watered every day, but not too much; different plants required different amounts of water and fertilizer. At first, he needed a piece of paper to remind him what plant got what, but he and Sheila had worked on this for so long that it was no longer necessary.

The garden wasn't just for show. The food that he grew here was what he ate. He didn't make anything to sell; this was where all of his vegetables came from. Paul still went to the store to get things he might need here and there, but as much as possible, he tried not to rely on outside food and power. He saw it as an important part of his independence.

Paul had been doing this for so many years that he couldn't remember how old he was. The only way he saw time passing was relative to how long ago Sheila passed, because he thought about her every day.

He didn't look back on his time with her in a grieving way any longer, however. He and Sheila had talked about the fact that one day, one of them would be left behind, and it was a fact they faced together with love and courage. It was beyond his belief that she was gone, in the beginning. But he knew better than to wish she was still here in the same way. She never left his thoughts, and her voice stayed with him. She was still here, but in new forms.

The two of them had lived a fulfilling life together. Now it was his job to tie up loose ends before he passed on himself. His will was already written, and he had a trusted lawyer who would take care of everything his children got when that happened.

It wasn't something he thought about often, though. It was only one thing on a long list of tasks he wanted to get done.

The most important on that list was what Sheila told him she wanted if she went first, and that was to make the garden more beautiful each day. It was a task that he took incredibly seriously.

Sheila knew how much she was asking of him whenever she gave him this wish. They had promised each other they would fulfill the other's wishes, but she knew that Paul was content keeping things simple. He wouldn't necessarily want the garden to be more extravagant than it already was. He found it more peaceful to leave things be.

But that wasn't the way Sheila saw it. She always wanted more. It made her restless to see it and feel like they weren't doing enough.

These days, the part of gardening Paul liked the most was the flower patch. The flowers used to be more of Sheila's responsibility while he took care of the plants they ate, but now that he tended them both by himself, it made him appreciate the flowers so much more.

He used to think it was a little less important to take care of the flowers. After all, they weren't eating them. But without Sheila here, he became more aware of the importance of having beautiful things around you. It made him feel better about being alive to see there was still beauty to be enjoyed, even when his favorite beauty was no longer here.

Paul was still thinking of the flowers as he drove to the gardening store. He had run out of seeds for his tomato plants, and to make the most of the next harvest, he would have to get more. Making this long drive on the highway wasn't something he wanted to do, but he had no other choice to get what he needed.

Since his house was out in the middle of nowhere, everything was a hassle to get to. He didn't much like creating more carbon emissions to get from point A to point B, either, but he didn't have another choice.

The long drives were something he saw to be worth avoiding, but there was no place he could get new seeds other than the gardening store, so he had to do it.

Sheila was the type of person who enjoyed car trips like this. She said it made her feel like a traveler; she wanted him to learn not to see all the little things in life as nuisances. You could see the good parts of the small, boring things in life, and you would appreciate life more as a whole.

He tried his best to adopt this way of thinking as he drove down the country road. Paul admired the land, thinking about how his and Sheila's garden compared to the others he saw.

There may have been a few that were bigger outside the farms, but he didn't think they compared to theirs — if only because theirs had more flowers.

He was glad he tried to see the good in this boring car trip because it helped him arrive at the store much more quickly. At last, he parked the car and went inside.

This was the kind of place outside his land. Paul was all right with going to. The store smelled like flowers and soil, things that were good and familiar to him.

It was one of the only places he frequented outside of his house, so he didn't feel as uncomfortable here as he did many other places. It also helped that there was usually no one else here besides him and the store owner, Andy.

He could tell there was something off about Andy today. The guy looked like he wanted to talk to him, but didn't at the same time. First, Paul put all the seeds in needed in a bag and went up to the counter.

"Nice to see you," he told Andy.

Paul waited to see if he had anything to say.

"You too, but I wish it was under different circumstances," Andy said, sounding more downcast than he had ever heard him before.

"What do you mean?"

"The store is closing. There isn't enough business out here," Andy said shortly. "There used to be more clientele, but they all moved out to the suburbs, and they don't come out here anymore. The people we do get aren't enough to keep us afloat. I'm afraid you found us on the last day we're open."

Paul's first thought was how heartbroken Sheila would be if she were here. She used to love passing half a day in this place, picking out flowers for their garden.

In the end, she only hand-selected a few, but those flowers always ended up being very special to both of them. The gardening store closing meant he wouldn't be able to relive those memories ever again.

This led to a change of plans for Paul, both for practical and sentimental reasons. First of all, he was going to buy a lot more seeds and fertilizers if this store wasn't going to be here anymore. He didn't know of any other place that was a reasonable driving distance from his house, so there was no telling the next time he could get these things. The sentimental reason was to see everything the store had to offer one last time. The more things he collected from the store now, the more memories he would be able to hold onto later.

After that, he gave one last goodbye and started his trip back home. Even though he was alone on the trip there and back, the trip back felt a lot quieter than the one there.

He thought to himself that there was some excitement to going to the store that he didn't fully appreciate; now that he knew he would never be able to go there again, he felt like he lost something he didn't even know he had.

Paul didn't have much of an internet connection at home, but he had to use the little service he had to find out where else he could get supplies for his garden. Most of his food came from gardening, so he did need to find out where his food was coming from. He was frustrated to find out there was nothing substantial within one hundred miles of his house.

Exercise

Daily Dose

TIME TO READ: 2 MINUTES

TIME TO DO: 8 MINUTES

A daily dose of meditation can help you enter a calm state. The best part about meditation is that it doesn't have to be difficult, and it can be quite pleasurable. The steps are simple, yet the rewards are great. Let your morning alarm be the signal to start your daily dose of calm.

1. Lie comfortably on your back in your bed. Notice your bed cradling your entire body. Place your hands over your diaphragm and begin to note the rise and fall of your belly as you breathe.

2. Imagine a clean black slate with just a small white dot in the center. Focus on the white dot.

3. While doing 2 + 4 breathing, bring your focus back to the clean black slate with the small white dot in the center. Focus on the white dot. Repeat four times.

4. While doing another round of 2 + 4 breathing, draw your attention back to your bed, cradling your body.

Imagine your body begging to become very light. Repeat four times.

5. While doing another round of 2 + 4 breathing, draw your attention back to your body. Imagine your body cradled in warmth. Repeat four times.

6. Now, count backward, slowly, from 100. End the exercise with a final round of 2 + 4 breathing.

Chapter 9. Home Sweet Home

It all started when Bobby Trainor noticed that old Mr. Jackson was not getting his groceries and was beginning to look frail and skinny. Bobby told Melanie, who was a close friend and who he actually had a crush on, about the situation. Then Melanie rounded up three of her girlfriends to join the now forming civic group, and there were five. Word got around, by the way, the school kid grapevine that there was a not-so-secret group that were helping old people and interest grew.

By the time the group expanded their operations, it was twenty-eight strong, and the only reason there were that few is that Bobby didn't know how to run a company or a large group of people as in this instance, because he was only 10 years old. They loved what they were doing, but they needed help, and they knew it. They met in an old barn on an abandoned farm on the outskirts of town. Everyone had a bike, and they all rode them to the meetings rain or shine.

They decided to call themselves "The Shadows" and the name stuck. One Sunday morning, Bobby's Dad was reading the Sunday paper and suddenly said, "Hey honey, it says here that somebody in this town is working small miracles for the old and the poor seniors. Bringing them food and bottles of water to make their lives better! How about that, eh? Now, who could be doing such a fine thing, I wonder?" he mused.

On Friday night, Melanie rode over to Bobbie's house and knocked on the door. "Oh, hello, Melanie," Bobbies Mom said, letting her in. "Bobby's up in his room. You know the way, go ahead on up and surprise him. I know he will love that." She said. Melanie bounced up the long staircase and burst into Bobby's room, but he had his back to the door and was wearing headphones. She snuck up behind him and quickly placed both or her hands around his head and over his eyes. He jumped violently, and the phones fell down across his eyes. "Hey, who's that?" he screamed and nearly fell off his chair. Mel laughed so hard that she actually did fall on the floor. They were becoming great friends and now had a huge band of brothers and sisters to run. They both liked that feeling.

"What's the plan, man?" Mel asked him. "Good, you're here. We have to call a meeting in the morning before lunch. Mr. Barker's cat is sick, and we need to figure out a way to kidnap him and get him the vets. Then we need to sweet-talk the vet into fixing him for free and get him back all good as new. You know that cat is all Mr. Barker has. He doesn't have any family to love and care for him. He probably doesn't even know this cat is sick." Bobby bemoaned. "Wait a minute. You said, "Kidnap." Don't you mean "Catnap?" she said, laughing again. "Ha-ha, very funny." Bobby countered.

The next morning just before lunchtime, most of the group members met up at the drug store in town and rode out to the barn together. The sight of all those kids riding their bikes in a pack like that; it must have looked like a bunch of young hoodlums. Who would have believed it if they only knew the truth?

Bobby opened the meeting after everyone had arrived and introduced the new mission parameters. Johnny Jenkins raised his hand because he had an idea. "I can get a big cat carrier from my sister and strap it on the back of my paper bike. I have a big strong rack on it so kitty will be safe. Where do we take him to anyhow?" Johnny asked. Little Susie Wilson stood up and announced, "My Daddy is a vet. Bet you didn't know that, did ya?" she asked. "Never mind that, Susie. Will he help us for free? That's what we need most right now." Bobby responded. "I will tell him we are going to do a favor for old man Barker. He'll help us if I ask him to." Susie told the group. "That's great, Susie," Bobby told her. "When do we do it?" asked Ron Goldman from over in the corner. "I think we'd better do it tomorrow as long as I hear from you Susie about your Dad helping us, okay? Call me as soon as you know, and let's just plan on meeting back here at noon tomorrow after that." Bobby announced. Everyone cheered, and the meeting adjourned.

"Bobby!" Mrs. Trainor called up the stairs. "Phone for you, kiddo," she hollered. Bobby came running down the stairs and grabbed the receiver. "Hello," he said. "Hi Bobby, its Susie, and I talked to my Dad. He said he would do it, so I'll see you at the meeting, okay?" Susie said. "Okay, Susie, good work," Bobby told her and hung up the phone. The day was getting late, and Bobby had already eaten his breakfast, so he told his folks he was going out and said goodbye. "You be careful out there, son," his Mom told him. "I will, Mom,

I love you!" he said with a loud voice. "Love you too, Bobby." She said and bent down to kiss him on the forehead.

Bobby waited for Susie to come by since she just lived down the street from him, and the two rode over to the barn together. At the meeting, Bobby asked for members to pitch in their ideas on what could possibly go wrong with the mission. Some of the kids called out stuff, but none of it would be a big enough problem to hold things up, so Bobby said. "Okay, guys, here we go. Operation Kitty Fix is a go!" and everyone cheered the way they always did and out the door, they went and rode off towards Mr. Barker's house to cat-nap his ailing kitty.

When they got there, they were out of luck. No cat anywhere to be seen, so they found spots here and there in areas around Mr. Barker's house where they could keep watch without looking like a bunch of hoodlums in training, casing the joint. Bobby was just about to call the mission when out of the partially open garage door came a limping and decrepit looking feline. "There he is!" Melanie said in a soft voice, and they all stood up at the same time. "Kenny, you go around back in case he bolts, Mel, you stand by the front gate in case he gets passed us and Ron, you're with me. Let's go!" And they moved out like the best trained Delta Force.

"We could have done this with one person?" Bobby said as he picked up the kitty and quickly slipped out of the gate and over to Ron's paper bike where the Pet Taxi was waiting. "The poor thing didn't even try to run, just stared up at me with his sad eyes and let me pick him up. Probably knew it could only get better for him. Cute little guy too." Bobby said as he zipped up the kitty carrier.

"All right, anyone who wants to go home besides Susie and Ron here is free to do so. Mission accomplished and now underway." Bobby announced. Nobody moved, so Bobby just sighed and got on his bike. When he and Ron started down the sidewalk, everyone began following. "Hey, wait a minute, guys. If you're all coming, at least, let's split up a bit. Half of you go to the other side of the street, so we don't look like a bunch of Sting Ray Renegades." Bobby yelled at them. "Susie, your Dad's vet is downtown, right?" Bobby asked. "Yep, it's on the corner of Main Street and 2nd. Avenue. When we get close, I'll take point, and you can follow my lead, okay?" Susie told them. "Sounds good." Bobby and Ron said at exactly the same time. They both fist-bumped, and Ron said, "You owe me a Coke!"

When they got close to town, Susie cranked up her pink machine and took over the lead just like she said. They all slowed down now, and she led them into an alley that runs behind all the downtown shops on the east side of Main. Soon, she turned into a small parking lot that only had two cars in it, and we all dismounted. "Is it all right if just you and Ron come in with me?" "Susie asked the crew. "Yeah, everyone stays out here and watch our bikes, and we'll be out in no time, okay?" Bobby told them. Susie, Bobby, and Ron, who was carrying the Pet Taxi, followed Susie into the rear door of the veterinarians. After ten minutes, they were back, and Bobby filled everyone in on the verdict. "They want to keep him at least overnight, maybe longer. They are going to do some tests and get his strength back up, but they said he would be just fine, so great job, everyone!" Bobby said to tired cheers all around. "Let's go home," Bobby said with a nod, and that was the end of another successful mission by the Shadows.

They continued doing missions and stayed friends for a few more years until the group splintered as things change the way they always do. Years later, Bobby married Melanie, and they had four kids of their own. Bobby stayed in the same house, and Melanie helped him to care for his aging parents as they slowly faded away. The kids in the neighborhood still rode "Sting Ray" type bikes and still looked to Bobby as though they were always up to something as they would go charging past his house every now and then on their way to who knows where.

Exercise   *Visualization*

If You See It, You Can Create It

TIME TO READ: 3 MINUTES

TIME TO DO: 7 MINUTES

Often athletes are taught to visualize their performance before competition. Many research studies have correlated how positive feelings and beliefs can positively affect performance. You can use visualization for yourself. For example, if you have a speech to give at school, visualize standing in front of the class; notice the students engaged in what you are saying. Confidently imagine how you remember all the talking points you have memorized. Notice how you speak in a calm, confident manner. Finish by imagining the class applauding at the end of your speech.

1. Set a timer for 7 minutes and get into a comfortable position.

2. Start the exercise with 2 + 4 breathing. Imagine a black room—so dark you cannot see your hand in front of your face.

3. Do another round of 2 + 4 breathing. Imagine accomplishing your goal. Once you have imagined it, determine the steps to accomplish this goal.

4. <u>Visualize it again</u>, as if you are running a movie in your mind, seeing every action step completed to accomplish your goal. Note the <u>sense of confidence</u> you feel in completing the goal.

5. End the exercise with a final round of 2 + 4 breathing. Repeat four times and then slowly open your eyes.

Chapter 10. The Sleeping Beauty in the Wood

Once there was an imperial couple who lamented exorbitantly because they had no youngsters. When finally, after extended pausing, the sovereign gave her better half a little girl, his greatness indicated his delight by providing an initiating feast, so excellent that the like of it was rarely known. He welcomed every one of the pixies in the land–there were seven by and large to stand guardians to the little princess, trusting that each might give on her some great blessing, similar to the custom of good pixies back then.

After the service, every one of the visitors came back to the royal residence, where there was set before every pixie adoptive parent a heavenly secured dish, with a weaved table linen, and a blade and fork of pure gold, studded with jewels and rubies. In any case, too bad! As they set themselves at the table, there entered an old pixie who had never been welcomed, because over a long time since she had left the ruler's territory on a voyage through delight, and had not been known about until this day. His glory, much beset, wanted a spread to be put for her; however, it was of normal delf, for he had requested from his diamond setter just seven gold dishes for the seven pixies aforementioned. The old pixie thought herself ignored and mumbled furious dangers, which were caught by one of the more youthful pixies, who risked sitting adjacent to her. This high back up parent, scared of mischief to the pretty child, rushed to conceal herself behind the woven artwork in the lobby. She did this since she wished all the others to talk first–so that if any evil blessing were offered on the kid, she might have the option to balance it.

The six presently offered their great wishes–which, in contrast to most requests, made sure to work out as expected. The lucky little princess was to grow up the most attractive lady on the planet; to have a temper sweet as a blessed messenger; to be splendidly effortless and charitable; to sing like a songbird; to move like a leaf on a tree, and to have each achievement under the sun. At that point, the old pixie's turn came. Shaking her head angrily, she articulated the desire that when the child grew up into a youngster and figured out how to turn, she may prick her finger with the shaft and bite the dust of the injury.

At this horrible prescience, every one of the visitors shivered; and a portion of the more gracious started to sob. The late cheerful guardians were practically out of their brains with misery. After that the savvy youthful pixie showed up from behind the embroidered artwork, saying merrily, "Your majesties may comfort yourselves; the princess will not bite the dust. I do not influence to modify the evil fortune just wished her by my antiquated sister–her finger must be pierced, and she will look at that point sink, not into the rest of death, yet into a rest that will last a hundred years. After that time is finished, the child of a lord will discover her, stir her, and wed her."

Quickly every one of the pixies evaporated.

The ruler, in the expectation of maintaining a strategic distance from his girl's fate, gave a declaration, restricting all people to turn, and even to have turning wheels in their homes, on the agony of moment passing. However, it was futile. At some point, when she was only fifteen years old, the ruler and sovereign disregarded their little girl in one of their mansions, when, meandering about at her will, she went to an old donjon tower, moved to its highest point, and there found an older adult so old and hard of hearing that she had never known about the lord's decree occupied with her wheel.

"What's going on with you, great elderly person?" said the princess.

"I'm turning, my pretty youngster."

"Ok, how beguiling! Allow me to attempt on the off chance that I can turn moreover."

She had no sooner taken up the shaft than, being enthusiastic and willful, she dealt with it so adroitly and thoughtlessly that the point punctured her finger. Even though it was so little an injury, she blacked out away without a moment's delay and dropped quietly down on the floor. The sick, terrified older adult called for help; in the blink of an eye came the women in pausing, who attempted each means to reestablish their fancy young woman, however, the entirety of their consideration was pointless. She lay, beautiful as a blessed messenger, the shading as yet waiting in her lips and cheeks; her reasonable chest delicately blended with her breath: just her eyes were quick to shut. At the point when the lord her dad, and the sovereign her mom observed her in this way, they realized lament was inactive all had occurred as the brutal pixie implied. In any case, they additionally realized that their little girl would not rest forever, however, following one hundred years, it was not likely they would both of them view her enlivening. Until that party time ought to show up, they resolved to leave her in rest. They sent away every one of the doctors and orderlies, and themselves pitifully laid her upon a bed of weaving, in the wealthiest loft of the royal residence. There she rested and resembled a dozing holy messenger still.

At the point when this hardship occurred, the mercifully youthful pixie who had spared the princess by changing her rest of death into this rest of a hundred years, was twelve thousand groups away in the realm of Marroquin. Be that as it may be educated regarding everything, she showed up expediently, in a chariot of fire drawn by mythical beasts. The lord was somewhat surprised by sight, however, in any case, went to the entryway of his castle, and, with a sad face, exhibited her his hand to plummet.

The pixie mourned with his magnificence and endorsed all he had done. At that point, being a pixie of extraordinary sound judgment and warning, she recommended that the princess, arousing following a hundred years in this old stronghold, maybe a decent arrangement humiliated, particularly with a youthful sovereign close by, to get herself alone. In like manner, without asking any one's leave, she contacted with her enchantment wand the whole populace of the castle aside from the lord and sovereign; tutors, women of respect, holding up house cleaners, men of honor ushers, cooks, kitchen-young ladies, pages, footmen–down to the steeds that were in the stables, and the husbands to be that go to them, she contacted each whatnot. Nay, with a kind thought for the sentiments of the princess, she even reached the little fat lap-hound, Puffy, who had laid himself down close to his escort on her mind-blowing bed. He, similar to all the rest, fell sleeping soundly in a minute. The very spits that were before the kitchen-fire stopped turning, and the fire itself went out, and everything became as quiet as though it were the center of the night, or as though the castle were a royal residence of the dead.

The ruler and sovereign having kissed their girl and sobbed over her a bit, however very little, she looked so sweet and substance left from the manor, giving requests that it was to be moved toward no more. The order was pointless, for, in one-fourth of an hour, there jumped up to around it a wood so thick and prickly that neither monsters nor men could endeavor to infiltrate there. Over this dense mass of woodland must be seen the highest point of the tall tower where the beautiful princess rested.

A considerable number of changes occur in a hundred years. The ruler, who never had a subsequent youngster, kicked the bucket, and his position of authority went into another illustrious family. So altogether was the narrative of the poor princess overlooked, that when the supreme ruler's child, being one day out chasing and halted in the pursuit by this imposing wood, asked what wood it was and what were those towers which he saw showing up out of its middle, nobody could answer him. Finally, an old worker was discovered who had heard his granddad state to his dad that in this pinnacle was a princess, wonderful as the day, who was bound to rest there for one hundred years until stirred by a lord's child, her ordained spouse.

At this, the youthful ruler, who had the soul of a legend, resolved to discover reality for himself. Prodded on by both liberality and interest, he jumped from his pony and started to drive his way through the thick wood. Incredibly the firm branches all gave way, and the appalling thistles sheathed themselves voluntarily, and the thorns covered themselves in the earth to allow him to pass. This done, they shut behind him, enabling none of his suites to pursue: at the same time, passionate and youthful, he went sharply on alone. The primary thing he saw was sufficient to destroy him with dread. Groups of men and ponies lay reached out on the ground, yet the men had faces, not passing white, yet red as peonies, and close to them were glasses half loaded up with wine, indicating that they had rested drinking. Next, he entered a vast court, cleared with marble, where stood lines of gatekeepers showing arms, however unmoving as though cut out of stone; at that point, dozed at their facilitate, some standing, some sitting.

Exercise

Connect Four

TIME TO READ: 2 MINUTES

TIME TO DO: 8 MINUTES

I don't know about you, but Connect Four was one of my favorite games as a kid. Four seems to be a good number for the brain. This is why 4 Square Breathing can be so calming. This exercise helps you reconnect to those feelings you avoid and allows you to move through them on a path of positivity.

1. Find a place to sit comfortably on the floor in a quiet room and set a timer for 8 minutes.

2. Focus your attention on your breath; if your mind wanders, bring it back to noticing your breath. Now, do a round of 4 Square Breathing.

3. Take a moment to find your inquisitive self. Scan your mind for awareness of unpleasant thoughts or emotions. Focus on these thoughts and emotions. Do another round of 4 Square Breathing.

4. Note the sensations arising in your body as you consider those unpleasant feelings or thoughts. Now, do another round of 4 Square Breathing.

5. Imagine a path lined with blue flowers and a bright light at the end of the path. Do another round of 4 Square Breathing.

6. Imagine entering the bright light at the end of the path and the sun warming your body. Now, do a final round of 4 Square Breathing.

Chapter 11. Autumn Dreams

Jenny shook her head in dismay as she looked at her child, sitting amid a veritable pile of candy wrappers.

A cold autumn breeze rolled in through the window and she got up to shut it.

"What am I going to do with you, kiddo? You are going to be up all night, bouncing off the walls with all that sugar! What was I thinking?"

Kirsty bounced on the bed, her gap-toothed grin fueled by entirely too much chocolate and marshmallow.

"Best Halloween ever, Mommy! I got, like, a hundred pounds of candy!"

Jenny laughed. The girl's enthusiasm was, if nothing else, infectious.

"I don't think quite that much, sweetie, but if you did, I'd box most of it up for next year!"

"Aww!" Kirsty wrinkled her nose. "I don't want to eat year-old candy!"

"I didn't say you'd have to eat it!" laughed Jenny.

"Maybe we'll give it to your father as punishment for letting you eat so much candy tonight!"

She sighed. Sometimes that man just did not think about things before jumping into them, and Jenny was left cleaning up the mess.

Kirsty giggled uncontrollably. "I bet he'd barf!"

"I'm sure."

"Do you think he would barf so much it'd fill up my candy bag, Mama?"

"Oh, gross, young lady! Let's not talk about such things before bed!"

Jenny reached out and lightly touched the tip of Kirsty's nose with her finger.

"Now, how am I ever going to get you to sleep in this condition? It's an impossible task!"

"What about a story, Mommy?"

Jenny put a finger to her lips and paused in thought.

"You know what? That's not a bad idea!"

She went to the self and picked up a well-worn paperback.

"No, not that one!"

Jenny's fingers glided over to a thin storybook.

"Nope! The big one!"

Jenny picked up the heavy book with the crackling cover.

"Yes!"

As she sat on her daughter's bed, Kirsty managed to bounce even higher in anticipation.

"This book is the best one, Mommy! The stories in it really come to life! Better than the other ones."

"Okay, this one it is, sweetie. Now lay your head back and let me find a good one."

Though its covers were weathered, as Jenny slowly turned the pages to find the right story, they felt glossy and new as when she was a kid.

"Let me see, let me see…."

A corridor of trees with leaves of red and gold arcing over a long road.

A lone branch had fallen in the road, a slender arm with a single thin shoot reaching away from the main branch.

It resembled a numeral "6," surrounded by falling leaves. As the mother and daughter watched, a few more leaves fluttered lightly to the ground.

"This is perfect for a brisk autumn night. We have got a toasty fire going downstairs. If you listen, you can almost hear its warm crackle…."

Glimpses of a sunset through the trees sprawled red, orange, and purple across the autumn sky.

The wind rustled the branches and fanned the leaves like crackling flames of red and gold that arced overhead.

Jaina felt as though she walked through a warm fire on the hearth itself.

The air was fresh but brisk with the fall sweeping through, and alive with the energy of changing seasons.

She breathed in deeply and the air smelled of pumpkin patches, sliced apples, tree sap, and the wood fires burning.

This time of year had a special resonance as summer gave way to winter and the changes that swept in before the leaves fell.

Nights like tonight were magic. A living dream.

She almost needed no sleep; to walk down the street on such a night was as invigorating as any night's rest.

As Halloween approached, the world came to life with creatures and half-glimpsed spirits rarely seen outside of this time.

The change was upon the world, in the rich scents that wafted through the air of baking pies, of sweet apples upon the trees, of cold drafts from distant lands, and fires upon the hearth.

Smoke drifted from the chimneys as she passed rows of houses. Orange light shone warmly in the windows against the darkening world. The faded blue scarf she kept wrapped around her neck trailed behind her in the breeze.

There was a field at the end of the street that Jaina had loved since she was a child. It was fenced off now; full of tall grass, and the derelict structures she had played with were long gone.

An old rusted tractor. Concrete chunks left from a house demolished long ago. A small hill with an old well.

She had made up so many stories about the lives that went unfolded in that place, the staging site for her adventures into distant castles and faraway lands, or lazy summer naps with her friends while the butterflies flitted slowly overhead.

In autumn, though, with a scarf around her neck and the change of seasons thick in the air, that field would serve as the gateway to many tales. As the butterflies changed through chrysalis, as the land changed during the autumn, so did her stories involve metamorphosis.

Jaina walked through the gap in the fence, her fingertips trailing over the cold metal links.

A shiver ran through her as she crossed the threshold, but not because of the cold metal's touch; because she had stepped across the gateway and into another world.

The grass rose around her steps, rippling in a sudden wind. Lights like fireflies appeared above trails that formed in the grass as hidden things scurried away.

A breath of wind spiraled around her, carrying with it leaves and memory: nutmeg and spice, a steaming hot cup of cocoa in the hands, smoke from the hearth fires, a soft but warm glow as the family huddled around the fireplace and shared stories. The perfect time of year.

Everything was transforming around her. Flowers opened in the field and then fell into slumber again.

Jaina knelt, hearing a strange sort of symphony in the growth and decline of the flowers.

A hum, like an old playground song, or the music her mother would play as they all danced between kitchen and living room, preparing a celebratory feast as fiery-colored leaves carpeted the yard. And there!

Jaina turned and she saw an aged barrel sitting there in the grass amid a cloud of fireflies and butterflies. Water sloshed in the barrel and the smell of fresh apples filled the air.

The sound of laughter and children's voices followed, and then she saw them, as though they had just sprung from the tall grass.

One of the children was her. Some of them stood on stepstools made of logs. The older ones were tall enough to stand.

They took their turns bobbing for the apples, splashing each other with cold water, giggling like mad.

Leaves of yellow and red swirled about the outside of the scene, like a shifting wall between dream and waking worlds.

Jaina smiled, seeing her older sister push her head into the water before she was ready.

Young Jaina came up sputtering, a leaf sticking in her matted hair. She had been so furious with Melanie that day!

Looking back at it, she laughed. What she would give to go back to that time when her biggest worry was her siblings tormenting her!

Turning to her right, Jaina saw another wall of leaves before her, which parted as she approached.

This time she stepped into a scene she remembered all too well: the night of her thirteenth birthday party.

Jaina's whole family had gathered in the front room with Grandma Gail; that was the last birthday she would ever spend with her grandma.

The old woman smiled at her over her glasses, saving the best present for last. Jaina remembered it well: the very scarf she wore around her neck.

Grandma had knitted it herself over weeks, in Jaina's favorite color: a cool blue, like the springtime morning sky.

She touched the fabric with her fingertips, still as soft as ever. Some of the colors had faded over ten years, but none of its comfort or warmth.

Grandma Gail had made it especially for those cooler autumn nights that Jaina loved to explore.

Gail looked up and met Jaina's gaze with her kindly smile. Jaina's heart leaped. A breath caught in her throat.

She stood transfixed as Grandma Gail raised a hand and waved to her.

Of all sitting in the living room, only young Jaina noticed, and she turned her head, searching for whatever her dear grandmother saw.

Young Jaina shrugged and turned back to her scarf, holding it up in the firelight. She wrapped it around her neck and beamed a smile as Gail turned back to her.

Both of their eyes lit up as they shared a special moment that would make one of Jaina's favorite memories.

The leaves shifted again and Jaina found herself walking beside a creek in a forest. Late afternoon sunlight shone through a golden-red canopy.

She remembered the area well: she had walked here often as a child, and later would bring the young man who would one day become her husband on their first tentative date.

This time she was walking behind herself, as a young Jaina balanced precariously walking along a log fallen across the creek.

Older Jaina smiled, knowing what was coming. "Watch your step!" she called, and it seemed like her younger counterpart heard something through the mists of dream and memory.

She paused, but it was too late. Her foot slipped on moss and she tumbled into the creek with a splash.

The water was bitter cold. Jaina came up spluttering and gasping for air, shocked by the frigid water. She laughed and clambered out onto the shore.

Of course, she had to go back to dry off next to a fire in the backyard, but first, she saw what had caused her to slip: a small cocoon hanging on the knot where she was about to put her foot.

She had noticed it at the last second and trying to avoid it threw off her balance.

Young Jaina found that the timing was more blessed than cursed, however: the chrysalis was beginning to hatch.

Exercise

Breathing through Lines

Exercise time: 10 minutes

Benefits: Raises awareness of breathing and assists in relaxation

MATERIALS: Paintbrush, watercolors, 1 sheet of 18-by-24-inch heavy-weight drawing paper, cup of water

1. Wet your paintbrush and choose a color to add.

2. Take a deep breath in through your nose. Hold your breath while you place your brush in the upper-left corner of the paper. As you exhale slowly, draw a wavy line.

3. Choose either the same color or a different color (don't forget to rinse your brush if it's a different color) and add it to your paintbrush. Take a deep breath in as you place your brush on the paper. This time, as you exhale, make a large circle with one breath.

4. Choose a color, but this time take short breaths in and out. With each exhale, make quick marks or ticks on the paper.

5. Pick a final color and breathe in deeply. Choose your own mark or symbol to add as you exhale.

Chapter 12. Forsaken Among The Forsaken

Hurry up Oden, else you'll be late for school Mr. Adams admonished as he stepped into his black Mercedes Benz ready to convey his only son Oden to school. Although he had made everything possible to ensure Oden improved academically, his son simply wasn't cut out for academic work. He was either too lazy to pursue his academic dreams or simply did not have the zest to do so. In a jiffy, Oden dashed out of the house dragging his schoolbag behind him. If there was a world competition for the best-dressed student, Oden would be up there among the top three if not the best dressed. His school uniform always sparkled, with seemingly unreplaceable ghetto lines.

In school, Oden wasn't the brightest. His teachers would often downplay his little efforts. His classmates didn't help matters also, they would often mock and make jest of him whenever he failed a question in class. Having been registered for extramural classes in his school, it is safe to conclude his parents wanted the best for him. Despite the frantic efforts put in by his parents to help him academically, it never translated into academic success for him.

Foden's mum was a full-time housewife. She stayed behind at home when her husband goes to work every day. Unlike her son, she was quite hardworking and committed to making the home a happy one. For over 12 years of her marriage, she literally sat at home every day performing household chores. It was one job she loved doing, but she was getting tired of repeating the same routine every other day. She wanted a new experience, a new dimension and a feel of what the professional world of business looks like. Although her husband initially debunked the idea, she persisted and she eventually got her way.

Oden was trying so hard to make an impression in class on a bright Tuesday morning. His teacher Mrs. West had put forward a question to the class. Mrs. West was their English teacher; though playful she could be very strict when necessary. Yes, you Oden she said as she pointed at Oden who had been raising his hands as an indication for his willingness to attempt the question. We stood up enthusiastically and gave the answer to the question. Whether he was right or not, he couldn't tell for a split second as the class was mute as if silence passed the classroom. Oden was left red-faced as his classmates rent the air with laughter. Obviously, it wasn't the laughter of approval or satisfaction. It was that of sheer mockery, downgrading, and morale-sapping. To Foden's consternation, his teacher was also visibly smiling. Among all his teachers, his English teacher would never openly laugh at him. At this point Oden felt completely alone, the laughter from his classmates was overshadowed by a grave feeling of solitude. Oden had never felt this dejected, he slumped back to his seat ashamed.

Mrs. West managed to curtail the laughter of the class and restored decorum, but the damage was already done. For the rest of the class, Oden was quiet. He didn't speak to anyone and no one bothered speaking to him. They rather cracked funny jokes about him and made a further jest of him. The school bell rang at about 3:00 p.m., which served as a mark of the closure of school activities for that day. With no friend to share his feelings with or console him at least, he stood alone in the terrace patiently waiting for his father's car to arrive. Before long, his father's car pulled over like a messiah as some group of students was walking towards his direction. He could only assume what they had in mind, perhaps to mock him again for his failures. At least this was not to be as he hurriedly raced to his father's car.

The time on the huge clock which hung on the wall opposite the entrance door of the sitting room was 6:05 p.m. Mrs. Adams would have been back by now, how come she isn't home yet? Mr. Adams wondered. Perhaps she has been stuck with work yet again. This was becoming quite unbearable for him. He never bought the idea of letting his wife work outside the home though she was a chartered accountant by profession. A few weeks ago, the dinner would have been ready by this time, but here he was, famished with absolutely little or no idea on how to conjure up the magic his wife usually did which led to those sumptuous meals.

Just as Oden and his father were struggling to piece together some food ingredients to make dinner, their savior arrived. It was Mrs. Adams looking all stressed out from her work. She couldn't wait to freshen up and rescue his husband and son from the kitchen. Left for her though, she simply would have taken a cold shower and toss herself on the bed.

As usual, it took Mrs. Adams wasted very little time in preparing the meal and goodness me, was it delicious? Of course, it was her trademark. On this occasion, however, Mr. Adams just wasn't happy not because of the food, but because of the recent lateness of his wife in closing from work. He was further bothered about his son's reluctance to hold a reasonable conversation since he came back from school. Mr. Adams didn't wait behind, as usual, to watch his favorite TV shows before going to bed. Instead, he went off to bed immediately after eating. This was something he rarely does and it was a clear indication that he wasn't happy.

Over the next few weeks, Mrs. Adams turned a new leaf, she no longer closed late from work. She prepared breakfast and dinner as at when due as usual. The Adams family was back to the happy home they used to be earlier saved for the woman doing a professional job and Oden being more taciturn. In the cool of a Friday evening, Mr. Adam decided to pay his wife a surprise visit at her office. Anyway, it was already a few minutes past her closing hours and it was weekend. He wanted to give her a surprise treat. Zoom, he went off as he throttled furiously on the less busy road that linked his house to his wife's working place.

On entering into the complex, he didn't find it difficult locating his wife's office. His wife was very good at description and has somehow managed to vividly describe where she worked. I believe I description of the building would be matched only by the architect himself who drew the plan. Mr. Oden was left disappointed as he knocked severally on his wife's office door with no response. Perhaps she had gone home earlier than usual. He decided to seize this rare opportunity to have a better look at the magnificent building as the staff was trooping out in twos and threes. He came across an office with its door slightly ajar, he was overtaken by over curiosity. All the office he had passed through were either locked or fully opened, why was this particular door slightly open? He decided to peep and satisfy his curiosity.

For the next few seconds, Mr. Adams simply stood there transfixed. He could not believe what his eyes have seen neither could his brain properly discern what was happening. Perhaps this was a symptom of blindness or he fell into a trance. He took out his white handkerchief which had been tucked away neatly in his back pocket and wiped his face to be doubly sure he wasn't going blind. After staring for a few more minutes he furiously dashed out of the complex as if chased by fierce masquerades. He cancelled every other plan he had for the night including the treat. There were more things more important than the others, he had to attend urgently to what had earlier left him bedazzled.

The tires of his car screeched as he furiously made a U-turn on impulse. He headed straight to one of his friend's apartment. He couldn't comprehensively share with his friends what his eyes had seen. He was still in shock and can't still get to believe that was what goes on in Cashmore Ltd where his wife worked. The essence of driving about 1km in the opposite direction of his house was utterly defeated as Desmond failed to make out exactly what his friend was saying. However, he resolved to calm him and down probably ask for a better explanation when he gets more calm and collected.

For the very first time since the day Oden was admitted to a hospital in an emergency, Mr. Adams failed to get back home. Both Oden and his mum were worried sick and attempts made to contact Mr. Adams ended in utter futility. Mrs. Adams's mind was slightly relaxed when he finally contacted Desmond and he told her Mr. Adams was just leaving his apartment. Why his husband would drive down to see Desmond on a Friday night was beyond her imagination. Still, she kept her fingers crossed and expected her husband to come back home all through the night, but that was not to be.

Oden was further plunged into the depths of loneliness and solitude in class. At some point, he contemplated suicide without his parent's knowledge, but he didn't know exactly how to go about it as he was still young. His teachers in school never helped matters at all. The last stroke which broke the camel's back came the day his principal mistakenly left him in detention from morning until school closing hours for performing poorly in class. He learnt absolutely nothing, completely abandoned in the principal's office at the mercy of the big bullies in school.

As they say, every disappointment is a blessing. This was the case of Oden that particular day. Instead of the big bullies who regularly piled on the misery on him to continue from where they left off, they rather sympathized with him and told him words of comfort.

Every one of them there had committed one grave offence or the other which violated the school's rules and regulations, but Oden to the best of their knowledge did nothing, but perform poorly in his academics. Soon Oden found solace in their company. Though he knew they were all members of a bad gang, he had no choice than to mingle with them. He had been forsaken for far too long by those who were supposed to have his back.

Exercise

Centering Meditation

Exercise time: 5 minutes

Benefits: Teaches meditation, fosters relaxation, slows down an active brain, and pulls focus to the present moment

MATERIALS: Phone or computer to play the Centering Meditation from

1. Sit in a comfortable spot and hit play on the meditation recording.

2. Once it starts playing, follow the meditation process.

3. Repeat this breathing exercise 3 times. If any thoughts come up, simply observe them and let them go.

Chapter 13. A Fishy Tale

Lure, check. Line, check. Pole, check. Everything seemed good for Paul's trip. The last little excursion of the summer, Paul wanted to catch the "big one" at Dreamer's Lake. While the size and description of the "big one" varied, people said that it was the biggest fish at Dreamer's Lake. Or maybe it was all a tourist trap. Either way, as soon as he was about to head out, he heard a gentle knocking at the door.

Paul opened the door of his quaint home to see Ryan at the door. Ryan was all dressed to fish, with a tackle box the size of a casket around his arms.

"All the other friends couldn't make it," Ryan said. "Work."

Paul let out a sigh. It was a battle getting the day off for him, but he thought that maybe Peter, Landon, and all his other friends could as well. Just one more trip with the boys was all he asked, but he assumed he'd settle for Ryan.

"Dang it," Paul said as he packed the rest of his belongings. The two hopped into Paul's truck, and with the gentle puttering of the truck leading the way, they were off.

Paul and Ryan did not say much during the journey to Dreamer's Lake. Occasionally, they'd look at each other, but besides that, they had nothing else to add to the conversation. Paul stared at the country roads in front of him.

The roads had that hypnotizing effect. Small twists and turns gave a bit of a mix-up, but otherwise, it was fields of corn and the occasional group of cows, munching on their hay and staring at the truck passing by. Someone's dog tried chasing after the truck, only to give up halfway.

Ryan looked out of the truck as well, at all the little country homes in front of him that were all lined up. Some were trailers, others were fancy houses. The scenery made Ryan yawn a bit.

"Tired?" Paul said.

"Yeah. Didn't get too much sleep last night. Was excited, you know? It's been so long since I fished." Ryan said.

Paul smiled. "It's going to be a good hour or two. You're free to take a nap if you wish."

Ryan laid his head down against the seat, and soon his eyes closed. Paul looked at Ryan, who already seemed to be in deep sleep somehow. Ah, if only the self-driving cars could come out. Both could get some extra Zs while the car gently takes them to their destination. But that technology seemed to be a few minutes away.

The truck continued to drift down the road, with not too much traffic blocking the way. Occasionally, he'd run into the Amish, but passing them was easy. As he passed the buggy, the trot-trotting of the horse filled his ears. He had to envy them a bit. Such a simple life they had. But he couldn't imagine the trip taking hours and hours on a horse-drawn buggy.

Ryan let out a snore, and Paul had to chuckle. Ryan was always the snorer of the bunch. Every time the crew spent the night, one of them wanted to put a giant cork in his mouth just to quiet him. It was like that sometimes.

About 30 minutes later, Ryan woke up, right after they hit a tiny bump. Surprisingly, he was quite energetic.

"So, what will you do if you catch the big one?" Ryan said. "Dreamer's Lake has a $1,000 reward. We could split it."

Paul chuckled. "As I keep saying, I don't think it exists. That reward has been around since we were children. It's just a little gimmick to get people to fish there. But I like Dreamer's Lake, as it is a decent fishing spot."

"Fair," Ryan said. "You're probably right. But in this boring life, you have to believe in something magical, even if it's a giant fish."

Paul had to chuckle at Ryan's remark, but he understood. Ryan had been through a lot in his life. He was sort of the black sheep of the group, coming from parents who always fought and put the blame on Ryan. Ryan grew up decently enough in spite of everything, but Paul could tell that Ryan had a deep sadness that he hid from everyone. It didn't help that, like everyone else, he had a mundane life and not much else going for him.

Perhaps a big fish could cheer him up. Even though it was supposed to be the thing of legends, he assumed that maybe there was a kernel of truth to it. Maybe there was a big fish, but it wasn't as big as people claimed.

After some time, Dreamer's Lake was right ahead. Sure enough, it was a bit packed. Cars lined up like little boxes across the parking lot. There was the parking lot, then a little park, and then the lake itself. He hoped that most people were there for everything else, not to fish.

Paul found a parking spot and stepped out, and they all double checked their gear to see if everything was in order. Everything seemed good to go for their fishing trip, and soon, they walked across the park. It was a nice day. That summer heat was still trying to cling on, but a cool breeze counteracted it. Couples lied down in the grass, staring at the nice clouds that drifted across the sky. Children played. In the wooded area, a photographer snapped a picture of a bird. Click. Click.

Paul had the temptation to join them, but with the sun setting earlier and earlier, he knew he had to act fast. Soon, they arrived at the boat rental place. They went inside, and the boat lady was behind the counter, her raspy voice moving through the area.

"What do you need?" she asked.

"Just a boat, please. Preferably a nice motorboat."

"Sorry, we're sold out of those."

"What about your lower ends?"

"Out of those, too."

"Then, what do you have?"

The swan boat's head bobbed back and forth as Paul and Ryan paddled across the river. Their movements stayed in a consistent rhythm, but even then, the boat moved quite slow. The swan glided across Dreamer's Lake in an almost trance-like movement, and it made both parties yawn quite a bit. This swan boat was meant for a relaxing trip, not one that was set on catching the biggest fish in the lake. Hopefully, the swan could do a whole lot more than gracefully glide across the water.

The real challenge was finding a spot to fish. Unfortunately, the lake was packed with fishermen and fisherwomen, and the two did not want any lines crossing, or any awkward stares as they fished. By the time they found a fishing spot, their feet exhausted themselves. The spot they found was right by a shoreline, located in a tiny corner around the lake. It was a little small, the chances are, they wouldn't find the big one here, but at least they could fish in peace.

They took out their fishing gear and began adjusting everything. They spooled the fishing line in a relaxing movement, and they made sure to hook their bait tightly around the hook. Then, there was a whoosh as they casted it into the water. The bobbers floated in the water, swaying back and forth as the ripples spread across the water.

The sun shined on these two fishermen as they waited for a bite. Until then, the two made some small talk. Talk that was small, yet had some meaning to it.

"How's the wife?" Ryan asked.

"She's doing good. I would have invited her, but fishing isn't her thing, you know."

"Ah. I'm talking to someone. Maybe it'll work out. She's a nice lady, but she still lives with her family and they treat her like a child. She wants to move in with me, but she doesn't have the money, and neither do I."

"That's silly. Watch out for those types. I'm sure she's nice, but you know."

The two exchanged some words back and forth, and then Paul's bobber went down. As it did so, Paul moved back a little, then started to reel it in. The fish did have a bit of fight in it, but it as it danced around underwater, its movements eventually stopped. Paul reeled it in. It was a nice catfish, the fish flopping a bit as the water dripped from its smooth skin.

"Well, at least we'll be eating well tonight," Paul said as he put the catfish in the bucket. It swam around, and the two resumed their fishing.

They kept fishing, and managed to catch a few more fish. Trout, blue gill, and a few other fish they didn't recognize went into the bucket. Many of Dreamer's Lake's fish weren't native, but imported from all around the world. This gave a bit of credence to the idea that the big one was a big lie.

Soon, they had a bucketful of fish, and the cracks of evening began to show in the sky. Soon, it would be time for everyone to go back. Once dusk hit, you'd get a good yelling at if you were still at the park. The last thing he wanted was to be treated like a teenage punk just because he was a little late.

Paul reeled in his line and sheathed his pole. "I think it's about time to get going," Paul said.

Ryan sighed. "Really? Just one more fish."

"All right," Paul said. "I'll watch."

The bob stood still in the water as the sun started to set. It was quite a beautiful sight to behold. In a way, it symbolized the end of summer and the beginning of a new season.

"I think it's about time to head out," Paul said.

"I guess so," Ryan said, and then he started to reel it back in. Suddenly, the bob dropped in the water like a cartoon character who discovered that gravity is a thing. The line began moving at a surprising pace, and Paul could tell that Ryan was using all his strength to keep the pole from flying out of his hands.

"It's a big one!" Ryan declared.

"No way," Paul said.

He looked down in the water. He could not see an outline of this fish, so he assumed it had to be deep down there. Knowing their luck, Ryan probably caught it on a log or something. However, Paul jumped in, grabbing the pole with his hands. He gasped at how heavy it was. Indeed, Ryan was holding on with all his might, and it made Paul gasp a bit.

The boat moved slightly, the swan boat going back and forth as they struggled. That thing was unstable enough already, but his made both parties gasp at the notion that the boat would probably be flipped over. Good thing they brought their life jackets, but this was the last thing they wanted.

Exercise

Gratitude Check-In

Exercise time: 5 minutes

Benefit: Increases positive effects on the nervous system

MATERIALS: Journal, pen

In your journal, list five things that happened today for which you are grateful. This exercise can be done daily, either when you wake up or going to bed.

Chapter 14. Mozart Moon

Home to famous composers, Beethoven, Mozart, and Bhram, it is no surprise that one of the most beloved traditions of Vienna is the opulent ball season. The height of which occurs January to February every year. The tradition reaches back to the 18th century as Imperial Austria celebrated and socialized annually in the Hofburg Palace, where the grand ball is still held to this day and where I will dance the night away just as the royals did for centuries before me.

You cannot arrive at a ball in any old vehicle, so for the occasion, we hired a horse-drawn carriage. Our steeds arrived at the hotel, both a stunning chocolate brown with braided mains. The carriage is sleek, black with gold accents, our chauffeur holds the small door open and extends his hand to help me into the carriage. Once settled under a soft blanket, we begin our journey to the ball. The streets of Vienna are filled with women in flowing ball gowns and men in tuxedos. Some are walking hand in hand to the palace, others have stopped for a meal and are in cafe windows watching us and other carriages roll by in the elegant transportation.

The courtyard of Hofburg Palace is ample, and we are greeted by towering statues of princes on powerful horses, a small army of cherubs, and Hercules himself at the front gate. The curve of the white marble palace glows with a golden bath of light, arches on the ground floor support a sea of columns above with the light accentuating every detail of the architecture. From our chariot, we float across the threshold of the palace and through the magnificent entrance. Marble floors stretch far into the distance. Every surface of the walls alternates from regal painting to ornate window frames, and from the painted ceiling hung two spectacular chandeliers sparkling high above. The ballroom is even more expansive, with viewing balconies on the second floor surrounding the dance floor and another softly painted ceiling decorated with several shining chandeliers curves above us.

We have the pleasure of being entertained with performances from debutants and professional dance companies before we have the honor of waltzing on the polished dance floor below. As the room begins to fill with more exquisite ball gowns and refined tuxedos, I begin to feel the fairy tale of living a royal life set in. The first performance is the debutante's dance, young couples attending the grand ball for the first time and executing a highly synchronized series of traditional dances to the harmony of the orchestra. The women are all dressed in long white dresses and elbow-length, satin evening gloves, and the men are in identical black and white tuxedos. In impossibly straight lines. They all move in unison to create a beautiful optical illusion as they turn and sway and lightly touch fingertips and bouquets. I am swept away by the fluidity and patterns made from humans moving in an alliance. To end their performance, they all dance an impeccable Viennese waltz. With white gloves held high in the air, and hundreds of identical small bouquets swirl around the floor, undulating to the rhythm of the orchestra. The debutante dance is followed by other highly choreographed dancers. Men in black tuxedos guide women in satin dresses, and ballet dancer's leap and spin. As a grand finale, two acrobats descend from the opulent ceiling strategically wrapped in long flowing white silks. They twirl in unison slowly down to the floor like leaves on a breeze.

Elated from the visual display of athleticism and grace, we make our way to the dance floor to do our best at emulating some of the skills we witnessed. We are grateful to find we are not the only couple with two left feet. We laugh with other couples around us and try dancing with different partners to little success. We do our best to be the replica of the Austrian royal family, but I can't help but make a quick running man move on the regal dance floor. We do our best at formal dancing up to midnight when the orchestra stops. Our hosts for the evening announce it is time for the traditional fin de siècle quadrille. This is the time of night that partners change positions with other couples in a long line that stretches across the room. As one, we march forward and back. We raise our arms; we spin and touch palms and twirl and change positions. We mingle and laugh with all the other guests in a well-mannered and impeccably dressed dance mob. When I do meet up with my partner again, it is our turn to swiftly dance back down the long line. We gallop past all the couples we had the pleasure of dance briefly with, and the smiles on every face is a memory I will carry with me for a lifetime.

After midnight more rooms open up, and we are free to explore. There is a chandelier room, dripping in the most decadent lighting I've ever seen. There are rooms designed for mingling with quiet music and a modern dance room with a DJ playing some of our favorite songs. We drink champagne and continue to make friends into the early morning hours. The night draws to an end. Still, we are not ready to finish our fairy tale, and new friends suggest a lovely place for breakfast. We eagerly accept the invitation. There is still some time before the cafe opens, so we slowly wander the plaza of the palace and the quaint streets that surround it. We take another shot at dancing the waltz and do surprisingly well on the sidewalks of Vienna. We pass by other guests, men with loosened the bowties, and women hold the lengths of their long skirts up to keep the hems from the light dusting of snow that has just started to fall as the sun rises across the city. The deep vibrant blue of the horizon sparks to life with an orange band of light, and the sun begins its daily waltz across the sky. The cafe is open, and we welcome a warm place to rest our dancing feet and continue to enjoy the fairy tale and company of our new friends.

Exercise

Power Affirmation

Exercise time: 10 minutes

Benefits: Creates a positive mindset and identifies real life events that support your affirmations

MATERIALS: Pencil, 1 sheet of 18-by-24-inch heavy-weight drawing paper, assorted markers

1. With your pencil, write an affirmation on the paper using bubble or block letters. An affirmation is a positive and short statement designed to help in goal manifestation. The key is to frame it as a confirmation of something that is true, even if you feel it's not quite true yet. Repeating an affirmation over and over will help it to become true.

Examples of affirmations include:

I am worthy.

I'm learning that it's okay to make mistakes.

I am open to discovering new meaning in life.

I love and accept myself the way I am.

2. Choose a marker and trace over the message. Hang the message where you will see it daily. Every day, say the affirmation out loud with deep conviction. Positive thoughts generate positive feelings and attract positive life experiences.

Chapter 15. The Sleep Blossoms

Let's begin by taking in some big, deep breaths. These breaths should be gentle and natural... Follow your own natural rhythm as you breathe in, and then out, over and over again. Just be present in your body and breathe for a few moments to yourself. In... And out... In... And out... With every breath that you take, imagine that you are getting lighter, and yet, as you continue to get lighter, you somehow manage to sink deeper and deeper into your bed.

Before you get too relaxed, it is time for you to get comfortable in your bed. Find just the right position for you; one where you feel safe, comfortable, and relaxed. It should be a position that lets you relax your entire body with ease that makes you feel better than you ever did before. This should be the position that you will sleep in. When you find it and you get into your comfy spot, just breathe...

Enjoy the moment...

Take a breath in, and hold it this time. Five... Four... Three... Two... One... And let it go, slowly and gently, through your lips. Imagine that you are gently blowing on a candle, not so strongly that the candle will go out, but just enough so the flame dances about. Take in another breath, right through your nose, and hold it. Five... Four... Three... Two... One... And exhale again, just as gently and just as slowly as before. Now, one more breathe. In... Five... Four... Three... Two... One... And out...

Now, as you feel yourself sinking deeply into your bed, deeper and deeper as you begin to relax, close your eyes if they are not already closed. Imagine for a moment that you are sitting right underneath a beautiful tree. The tree is a cherry tree, and it is in bloom. The cherry tree is right next to a quiet stream that is passing by, and you move, in your mind, toward the tree. You can smell the soft, gently sweet scent of the delicate cherry blossoms, and you sit right underneath it. Your back, in your mind, rests against the tree's strong trunk, and you feel supported. You know that this tree will hold your weight and it will keep you there for as long as you would like to be.

As you sit underneath this cherry tree, you watch the stream. It is not a very big stream, nor is it deep, but it flows by gently. Imagine its sound as it flows past you, gently babbling away. You sit there and listen to the babbling of the stream and you breathe in and out, enjoying the relaxing, calming scent of the blossoms and sinking deeper into relaxation.

Feel your body sink deeper into your bed, and imagine that the relaxation is moving everywhere throughout your body, leaving it feeling as warm as you like. Feel the bed providing you with the support, gently conforming to your body, but still holding you up where you need to be, keeping your back nice and straight, just like you need. Feel that same support that you felt from the tree reminding you that you are sturdy and safe and strong.

Then, move back into your mind, retreating back to that image of you underneath the cherry tree. You sit there, tall and supported and relaxed, and then a breeze passes by. It is not a strong breeze at all; the leaves on the tree and the blades of grass underneath you barely quiver as it washes over them, and yet suddenly, you see a cloud of pink pass you by. But, upon closer inspection, it is not a cloud at all; it is a wave of pink cherry blossoms that have been moved from the tree! The blossoms slowly drift downward, falling into the water all around you, and then you notice something; the stream is not very powerful, either. The blossoms drift onto the surface of the stream and slowly and lazily drift away, spinning in slow circles as they are moved.

The stream in front of you is your train of thought, and all of the petals that have just fallen into the water are all of your tensions and worries that you have built up over the day. They are all of the things that have brought you down throughout your day. They are the frustrations, the fears, the arguments, the sadness, and anything else that weighed heavily on your mind as you worked throughout your day. The petals, as pretty as they are, represent all of the things that are keeping you awake as you lie in bed, trying to sleep... And they all need to wash away before you can sleep.

Watch each petal as they drift away. Pay attention to each one for a moment or two as you work through this. The first petal that you see, lazily drifting through the water's slow currents, is the anxiety surrounding your day. You must watch that anxiety, waiting for it to flow down the stream. You might feel the urge to pick it up or to hold onto it or to try to force it down into the water to drown it, but that will not work. The only way to be rid of it is to let it pass you by as slowly and as gently as possible. The only way that you can really help it along is by letting it go and by breathing.

You take in a great, big inhale, breathing in that soft scent once more. Hold it... Five... Four... Three... Two... One... And exhale it. Let that air out, and watch as your anxiety goes around a bend in the stream, out of sight and out of mind. The water in front of you is clear... and then you see more petals coming your way as well. Just like before, the only way that you can help these petals to pass is to help them to go on their own without any resistance on your part. You must simply watch as they slowly and quietly drift away.

The next petal that drifts in front of you is the petal that holds your fear. Remember, your fears are a little bit different from your anxiety; your anxiety is there before the fear. The fears are the thoughts that you have that scare you, and they must also be released into the stream to keep on flowing and to stay away.

You breathe again, deeper this time if you can. In... And hold it... Five... Four... Three... Two... One... And exhale. You notice that, with that exhale, the petal gets a little bit further away from you. It drifts a little bit further down the stream. You take another big, deep, diaphragmatic breath, breathing in... And holding it... And out... And again... And again...

And after you have breathed in and out long enough, the petal of fear, too, drifts away. It disappears around the bend, leaving your mind a little bit freer for a little bit longer.

Now, another petal drifts in front of you—three, actually, and you realize that they are sort of stuck together by something sticky, perhaps sap or nectar or something. These petals are your tension, your stress, and your worry. They are a bit heavier than the other petals, and they go a bit slower as they go past you. They get stuck on a small plant in front of you, simply sitting there without anywhere to go, and as the petals are stuck, you, too, are weighed down by your stress, your tension, and your worry. You need to release them, too, and the only way to release them is through breathing deeply and slowly to fill your body with relaxation to force those feelings out and allow you to feel other feelings instead.

You breathe in... and out... In... and out...

You notice that, in bed, you are starting to feel heavier than ever as you sink into your bed. You feel like you and your bed are inseparable, and that the deeper that you sink, the more in sync you feel with your body and your mind. You are comfortable in these feelings. You enjoy the sensations that you feel within your body, and you thrive on them.

Soon, as you return back to your cherry tree, you see that the petals have become dislodged, and they are floating away from you. You can see them disappear out of sight, and therefore out of your mind for the night.

You realize that, as you sit against the tree, you feel quite relaxed. You are enjoying your current feelings, and you feel like your heart is floating just as daintily and gracefully as the blossoms as they fell... But then, you realize that there are many more pink spots within the stream that is your mind. They are spots that will have to be cleared out, too.

On closer inspection, however, you notice that the pink that is left are all whole flowers. They are not blossom petals at all; they whole blossoms are there in their entirety, looking beautiful as they lazily float on the gentle stream. These are your sleep blossoms; they are here to help guide you to sleep. You will look at each one during your deep breaths, and each one will bring to you more and more feelings that will help you become more relaxed and sleepier than ever. With every blossom that passes by, you will feel more and more relaxed. You will feel sleepier and sleepier... And you may even drift to sleep as they go by.

You breathe in... And the blossom drifts in front of you. This one brings with it the feeling of peace that you feel in being chosen by a young puppy or kitten that wants to cuddle with you to sleep. It is that peace of heart and that love that you feel when the baby animal curls up in your lap, entirely of its own volition. It is that feeling of being sought out and chosen to bring comfort to someone else, unprompted. It is warm... It is pleasant... It is relaxing... And the blossom drifts away.

Exercise

The age-old question, "Who am I?" comes to mind when you work on a self-portrait. An image of yourself can bring revelation and insight. Your true self will come through as you create your self-portrait. The details you depict and the colors you choose are an extension of you. Before you get started, ask yourself how you would like to be remembered and how you think others see you. Also contemplate your best qualities.

BENEFITS:

Increases personal reflection and self-awareness

Exercise time:

1 hour

MATERIALS:

- Photo of yourself
- 1 sheet 18-by-24-inch heavy-weight paper
- Mod Podge
- Acrylic paint
- Paintbrushes
- Cup of water

STEPS:

1. Choose an image of yourself from the past or present. Make a photocopy of this image, either in black and white or color.

2. Apply a layer of Mod Podge to your paper.

3. Place your image on the Mod Podge, and then layer Mod Podge on top of the photo. Allow it to dry for 20 minutes.

4. Use the paint to add color and emotional expression to your art.

Chapter 16. The Lovebirds

Once upon a time, there was a princess, she was beautiful and had beautiful long locks and beautiful blue eyes.

Not really that you would say, "She can't get a prince."

And yet she didn't get a prince. Because there was a crisis going on in the country, and the princes didn't have that much money left, so they didn't even go to the wedding, of course.

So that beautiful princess was waiting for the crisis to end. And that only lasted and lasted. She was a bit tired of waiting. One day, however, a large giant came by and stole the princess from her balcony as she watered the flowers on her balcony. Hopping in his big Kinking hand, he plucked her as if she were the flower from her castle balcony and tucked her into his pocket like that. Now that felt nice, so the giant walked home quickly, with his new acquisition.

The princess was pretty scared and screamed that it was a sweet delight, but of course, nobody heard her in that significant giant record. Finally, she fell asleep against his warm pocket.

After many hours, they arrived at his huge castle, which he had once stolen from a king in a nearby kingdom. He had eaten the king and his family and said, "Now this is my kingdom and my castle."

And so, it went in those days.

Arriving at his big castle, the giant put the princess in a golden cage. It was a giant birdcage, with two large food bowls and a swing in the middle. The princess climbed directly into the rhythm because she liked that.

She rocked that it was a sweet delight all day long, and she even started singing. Satisfied, the giant looked through the bars at his beautiful princess, stopping some princess sowing seed in the manger. But after weeks of rocking and singing, the princess also wanted something different, and she got bored.

She wanted to get out of the cage and of course, home. So, she started to grumble against the giant. Now, if the giant could not stand something, then it was against grumbling princesses.

He felt like a giant bull. With irritation, he lit a giant joint to get out of the routine, but the princess became nauseous with that little odor and gagged in her golden cage. 'Stop that on you! With that dirty smell. Hop out, "she shouted. She raised her fist against the giant.

The giant is now pretty stoned, looked at her bored, "say, child, what do you want?"

"I want a prince, a real one!"

"And a very nice one too," she muttered.

"Okay," said the giant, filling the food bowls again and pulling out.

It took a few days for him to come back, and the princess sobbed on her little swing in the cage. Her nose is red with tears and sniffles.

But the big door opened and there he was again, a real prince with a sword hung on his finger, with which he tried to prick the giant. The giant smiled at himself and put the angry prince in the golden cage with the princess.

The prince was blazing, "filthy rotten," he sneered, "come here if you dare!" The princess took a relieved breath, look at it, finally a real guy with guts!

She flew the prince around his neck, out of her swing, and the prince did not know how he had it, actually the beauty of a princess in a golden cage.

He stammered in surprise, "What have you got a red nose?"

"Yes, it's because I had to cry," the princess said happily.

"What beautiful eyes you have," the prince said then. "Yes, that's because I'm a princess, of course," the princess laughed.

"Okay," said the prince, "that makes sense, of course," smiling, he put one arm around her waist and looked deep into her beautiful eyes.

"How long have you been here," murmured the prince?

"Oh, a few weeks already," smiled the princess.

She also had beautiful lips, the prince thought, and they began to kiss each other.

The giant looked at all of this and thought it was beautiful, clapping his big giant hands.

Look at his lovebirds might have gotten a boy he could eat!

The prince's sword settled on the bottom of the golden cage, and they sat there, kissing for a few minutes.

Immediately in love, just like that, the giant had found a good prince.

How did he manage this?

But the big question was, how did they get out of that cage?

But they came up with a plan together.

One day the prince said to the giant: "Hey giant come here."

The giant came rushing because he had smoked another big joint and was as slow as a canary, of course.

"What issuer dude," murmured the giant dazed?

'Well, my princess is having a baby, and we want to make a nest now and then. Do you have some nesting material for us? "

"Sure," the giant said happily. "Hmm, human babies, he loved it so much." The giant gathered some straw and hay together, and an old clean handkerchief could also get rid of it.

For example, that day, the princess tore the mega large handkerchief to pieces, and the prince stuffed a nest into one.

It had become a beautiful and large nest where the two of them could sleep comfortably. And they did that, sleeping together. They loved each other a lot, and especially in difficult times, this sometimes brings people closer together.

The next day, the prince threw the nest upside down, and the princess sat down under it, the prince climbed close to the golden cage door and called the giant, "Giant?"

Giant, come here? "

The giant just came out of his big giant bed and shuffled at the cage, "what is it again," he asked with a morning mood; you get that. With giants that blow. "Our nest has fallen, can you put it up?"

The giant went into the cage with his giant hand and wanted to lay the nest upright, but suddenly the princess stuck him with the prince's sword in his hand.

"AUWWWWWWWW," echoed through the castle. The prince jumped out of the cage, and the princess climbed quickly.

The giant was crying like a child, with a finger in its mouth.

They quickly ran away through the castle and found their way out.

Together they ran through forests and over heathland, and finally, they arrived safely at the prince's castle.

"Come, my dear, we are finally home."

"Say that," the princess laughed happily. They flew into each other's arms, and they lived happily ever after.

Exercise

A mind movie is a snapshot of the life you desire. It allows you to see life in the present, as if what you have imagined is already in your possession. Consider positive events from your current life that have brought you joy. What if you could manifest similar experiences? It's important to view your mind movie daily to bring about good feelings and add clarity to what you desire out of your life.

BENEFITS:

Identifies strengths, imagines positive experiences, and manifests future events

Prep time:

10 minutes

Exercise time:

50 minutes

MATERIALS:

Computer

PowerPoint software

STEPS:

1. Take 10 minutes to brainstorm what you desire out of life.

2. Type one of your desires onto a PowerPoint presentation slide.

3. Find an image to match that desire and place it on the next slide.

4. Repeat the process to create several slides using your desires and images. You can use images from the Internet as well as from your own life.

5. Consider adding your favorite song to the presentation.

6. Watch your presentation in slideshow mode once a day.

Chapter 17. Floating Forever Downstream

The mountains stretch forever, in every direction. Civilization exists in some other place, and some other time. Here, now, it is only you, and you are flowing downstream, endlessly, on a raft of your own design, with blankets, and nothing to occupy your thoughts or your feelings besides your surroundings, and the sensation itself, of floating, forever, lackadaisically, relaxed, at a snail's pace, down this stream, this vein flowing through the heart of the earth, all the blood of life passing through, effortlessly, slowly, from the heart and back to it. You do not remember when or where you started, and you have no idea when or where it will end, just that it will be a very, very long time, and a very, very, very long way away. The repetition of the scenery hypnotizes you, yet, somehow, each new area is so pleasantly new in some subliminal way, you feel endlessly entertained, like some enchanted treadmill of the soul, you could watch these repeating trees, huddled together, endlessly, for the rest of your life, and you would be perfectly content. Each new grouping of trees, each new formation of rock you pass, each shore, so unique in its own way, feeding your soul in a totally sustainable cycle. You become accustomed to this repeated stimuli, and it creates a new homeostasis in your mental being of perfect satisfaction. The breeze is steady, soft kisses on your exposed skin, and the flow of the river is steady, yet wild, in a pleasant, relaxing way. There are swoops and sways, and each stretch of the river is totally different from the last, yet so familiar, and so endless, and so assuring in its repeated, steady flow downwards. Sometimes the river is more wild, pushing you up and down like little hills, little waves knocking around your raft, surfing along them, wondering if it is possible you could be flung off, yet you never are, so you become more and more relaxed, realizing your comfort level, and that this little raft can take a lot from this river, and that this river will never give more to the raft, and you, than either can handle. Then, sometimes, the river is more calm and peaceful for long passages, almost as if it is going to bring your raft to a standstill, yet these passages are just as entertaining and life-affirming, for they allow you to take an even great measure of the immense scenery, the trees, the shrubbery, even the sky above you, as well as yourself, and your internal scenery, your life, and your body, your blood and your soul. On one of these long, peaceful passages, you spot a family of deer, and, taking advantage of the calm river before them, they cross right in front of your raft. You say hello to them, and they look at you, and it humbles you to see them so comfortable with your presence, it makes you very happy and you feel very much as if you are totally at one with the nature. You feel almost as if you are a part of this river, like a branch, having fallen of a tree a long ways back, being taken down the river wherever it may go, to be digested by the earth somewhere along the way, taken in, absorbed, and given back in some new form, somewhere back up the road, of space, and time. The perpetual cycle of things is very apparent to you here, on this trip. This river itself is almost as the river of time. Down and down, it keeps going, never ending, and an endless forest surrounding it, endless places for it to go. As it goes, it carves a path, and the path becomes new things, and life is given along the path, by the waters, and life is taken down the path, by the waters, and brought elsewhere. Where it goes, nobody knows. For infinity, down the river, down, down, and down, into the ocean, then, somehow, by a long journey of will, back again, back to the top of the mountain, only to, eventually, succumb to the river, relaxed, letting the river take it down, sleeping, down back to the bottom. So is life, so is the nature of all things. Here, where you are, now, you are on that journey back to the bottom, back to the well. On this journey, it is your job only to relax. All the work is behind you. Now the river is doing all the work that is to be done for you, by the flowing of the water, by time itself. By the end, you will be at the bottom, and you will be placed sweetly back into the ocean, if there even is an end, which, to you now, is unknowable. As you are not consciously aware of the beginning, you are also not consciously aware of the end, only the nature of all things, and the knowledge that eventually, somewhere along the line, everything must end, and return to wherever it is that it came from. Still, in your state, it is merely for you to focus on the here and the now, and the floating, forever, downstream. Day turns into night, repeatedly, and the noises from the forest take suit. The light green fauna of the day turns into a dark web of mystery at night. You see glowing eyes peering from the trees, and here low growls, and footsteps, wild beasts stalking in the night, as you float endlessly past. The rumbling and grumblings occurring within their natural ecosystem, all throughout the endless forest, apart from you, as you take passage, a passenger, down the stream, through it all, and away. Days pass by and you stare, fixedly, allowing the passing forest to warp into some hypnotizing blur. The noises of the wild come upon you; as if the embodiment of the forest is some spirit, besides you in the raft, whispering playfully to you, great, grand nothings. You laugh, laugh at a joke being told to you by the Great Spirit, and you yawn. Your eyelids become heavy, as another transition into the dark mystery of the night begins, apart from you, as you journey through life, down the stream, relaxed, on your back, body rested, and comfortable, and totally still, feeling for eternity the soft rocking of the raft on the infinite waters, the stream of consciousness flowing forever down the mountain. You close your eyes, and listen to the cooing of the forest, and rustling of the leaves in the wind, easing your mind into a higher state of consciousness, away from itself, up as you are down, into dreams.

Exercise

Mindfulness?

If you pay attention to what your mind is doing, you'll notice two strong tendencies:

The mind focuses on things other than what is happening right now. Most of the time we're thinking about events that have already happened or that might happen in the future. Thus, our well-being is often affected by things that have little to do with the moment in which we find ourselves.

The mind continually evaluates our reality as good or bad. It does so base on whether things are working out the way we want them to. We try to cling to circumstances we like and push away those we dislike.

These tendencies are part of what it means to be human. They can also cause us problems and needless suffering. Focusing on the future can lead to worry and anxiety, most often about things that will never happen. Ruminating on events from the past can lead to distress and regret about things that are no longer in our control.

In the process, we miss the once-in-a-lifetime experience that each moment offers. We don't really take in the people around us, the natural beauty of our surroundings, or the sights, sounds, and other sensations that are here right now.

Our constant and automatic effort to judge things as either for us or against us also creates unnecessary pain. We often end up resisting things we don't like, even when such resistance is futile. A perfect example is raging against the weather—no amount of cursing the rain will make it stop, and we'll only frustrate ourselves in the process.

The practice of mindfulness offers an antidote to both of these habits.

Chapter 18. Honolulu Dreams

Before you begin your bedtime story, you will first need to center yourself and still and calm your mind. This part of the guided meditation will be very important to your nightly practice because without starting from a place of stillness, it will be difficult to let yourself completely engage with the story and get the maximum benefit from each carefully crafted guided meditation.

Guided meditation is most effective when a person has strong visualization skills. In order to develop these skills, it is important to practice using the imagination to create a vividly detailed image.

Begin by imagining yourself exactly as you are, standing in a small, white room. There is nothing in this room but you and the white walls, white floors, and white ceilings. There are no windows and no doors. Just you, completely surrounded by white.

Now, picture yourself looking up at the plain white ceiling. The ceiling is completely bare until you decide to place navy blue polka dots across it. Now, there are navy blue polka dots across the white ceiling. See the navy-blue polka dots stretch clear across the ceiling and let them begin to cascade down the walls. Now the walls in the room you are in are also covered with navy blue polka dots.

You are now standing in a room that has a white floor and has navy blue polka dots on the walls and the ceiling. You are surrounded by navy blue polka dots. Look down to the floor and now, picture the floor covered in navy blue polka dots. Everywhere you look, navy blue polka dots!

Now, you are going to change the color of the navy-blue polka dots. Instead of navy blue, the polka dots are now a butter yellow. You are in a white room with butter yellow polka dots on the floor, walls, and ceiling. Nothing but butter-yellow polka dots, everywhere you look.

The purpose of this exercise is to use your brain to create vivid mental images from word prompts. The clearer your mental images are, the more you will get out of guided meditation. The practice of visualization is a powerful tool that is often included in meditation practices and can be used in a variety of ways.

Picture yourself standing on a long, sandy beach. The sand is white and glitters in the strong Hawaiian sun.

You are on the Hawaiian island of Oahu, and you are at Waikiki Beach. You look out across the aquamarine water of the Pacific Ocean, and you take a moment to take a long, deep breath in of the fresh, salty sea air.

You walk along the beach, the cool waters of the Pacific Ocean gently caressing your bare feet. You smile as you watch the many children that gather in this particular area of Waikiki to play in the shallow, calm waters. They gather here because there is a stone wall that was built here that creates a naturally protected lagoon, and families like to come here to enjoy the fresh saltwater without fear of the waves.

You are making your way towards this wall now. The wall isn't that high up when you first enter on to it. It looks a bit like a long boardwalk, and you enter from the sand. You continue walking on this wall, and the ocean becomes further and further away underfoot. Finally, you reach the end of the Waikiki Wall and you are standing under the small pavilion at the end.

The pavilion offers a bit of shade from the intense Hawaiian sun, and you revel in the cool sensations of both the shade on your exposed skin and the cool stone under your bare feet. Out here, you can hear and see the waves of the Pacific Ocean as they roll in on the other side of the wall. You close your eyes for a moment and listen. The wave's crash in and out with a familiar regularity that feels and sounds like stability. Even in this wild and unpredictable natural element, there is still stability to be found here.

You sit on the edge of the Waikiki Wall and look down. On one side of you is the protected lagoon, where small children are able to play without worries of waves and sharks. On the other side is the unchecked raw power of the Pacific Ocean, where the waves roll in and roll back out, without manmade protection.

You are listening still to the comforting and familiar sounds of the waves as they roll in and roll back out, crashing against the natural shore and the manmade Waikiki Wall. You feel safe in the knowledge that something as wild and free can be both counted on for some semblance of regularity and can also be contained to a certain extent. When the tide comes fully in, this Waikiki Wall will be useless, but it does the job for now, and the many people enjoying the peaceful manmade lagoon here appreciate it for what it is.

Life can be like that, right? There are things in life that are impossible to control, but there is always something that a person can do that can make them feel like they have some sort of power in the situation. Sometimes all you need is to find the thing you can count on, like the Pacific Ocean waves as they crash against the shore at Waikiki Beach in Honolulu.

Let your mind drift back to your present reality. Take a long, deep breath while counting to three: 1 – 2 – 3 and back out 1 – 2 – 3. Again, deep breath in 1 – 2 – 3 and back out 1 -2 – 3. Do this as many times as you would like, letting your mind slowly come back to your present circumstances.

Remember, even in the midst of something that you cannot control. You can still find something comforting within the unpredictability. Can you think of any time in your life where having accurate expectations helped you to deal with something out of your control? Your personal examples do not need to be grandiose or complicated- they just need to be yours. Let yourself remember the lessons of the Waikiki Wall in Honolulu, Hawaii, and perhaps you may find yourself back there in your dreams...

Exercise

We explored the powerful and far-reaching effects of simply being fully in our experience with greater openness. Formal practices like yoga and meditation complement moments of mindfulness in our everyday activities. We also saw how these practices have been integrated with CBT and shown to effectively treat many conditions. If you're working on behavioral activation and/or changing your thoughts, mindfulness principles dovetail perfectly with those practices. Subsequent we will include practices from all three pillars of CBT.

It's normal to have misgivings about mindfulness, which often are based on false impressions of what the practice is about. If you're ready to try mindfulness for the first time or want to deepen your practice, I invite you to take the following steps:

1. Begin to notice what your mind is up to during your day. Is it focused on the past, the present, the future? Is it opening to your experience or resisting? Take care to just notice, letting go as much as possible of judging what your mind is doing.

2. Choose a small number of activities to practice mindful awareness during your day, using the six principles.
3. Begin a meditation practice. If meditation is brand new to you, start with just a few minutes a day
4. Reading this on mindfulness can reinforce the concepts from this and contribute to a robust practice.
5. Practice incorporating the principles of mindfulness into behavioral activation and retraining your thoughts. For example, bring enhanced awareness to your planned activities to maximize the enjoyment and sense of accomplishment.

Chapter 19. Lisa Bakes A Cake

Tonight, we are going to enjoy a lovely story about my good friend Lisa, and the cake she baked with her dad!

This cake story is going to be so much fun; I know you will love learning about how to bake a cake with Lisa.

Before we can sink into a lovely story, though, we have to make sure that you are comfortable and relaxed enough to listen!

Make sure you have done your entire beautiful bedtime routine and that you are ready to lay completely still and listen to this story.

If you have not already, get a sip of water, say goodnight to your family, and get cozy in your bed.

Then, we can start with a nice and easy breathing meditation to help you calm your body down so that you can have a great sleep tonight.

 Are you ready?

Let's begin with the simple breathing meditation.

For this meditation, I want you to imagine that you are holding a balloon in front of your face.

Can you do that for me?

Great!

Now, let's imagine that you are going to take a nice, deep, slow breath in through your nose, and then you are going to blow out through your mouth as if you were trying to fill the balloon up with air!

Starting now, breathe in nice and slowly through your nose, filling your lungs up with air.

Now, breathe out through your mouth as if you are trying to fill a balloon up with air!

Perfect, let's do it again.

Breathe in slowly through your nose, and now breathe out through your mouth to fill up your balloon.

Breathe in slowly, filling your lungs all the way up, and then exhale through your mouth, filling the balloon up with air.

Breathe in slowly, and once again breathe out filling up the balloon.

One more time, breathe in slowly through your nose, filling your lungs all the way up with air.

Now, breathe out through your mouth filling your balloon all the way up with air!

Perfect!

Now let's imagine that your balloon full of air floats away into the night sky, leaving you relaxed and ready to enjoy a wonderful story and a good night's sleep.

Goodbye, balloon!

One day, Lisa's dad told her that her mother's birthday was coming up!

Excited, Lisa started planning out what she could do for her mother's birthday.

Lisa was only eight years old, so it was not too easy for her to go to the store and pick out a lovely present to celebrate her mom.

So, she asked her dad to help her pick out a present and to help her bake a cake for her mom.

Of course, her dad said yes, and so in the week before her mother's birthday, Lisa's dad took her to the mall to pick out a present for her mother.

While there, Lisa picked out a beautiful silver necklace that said "mom" on it and had a heart shape around it with three rhinestones in the heart.

Lisa brought it home, wrapped it up, and hid it in her closet so that her mother would not find it before her birthday.

On the day of her mother's birthday, Lisa and her dad took to the kitchen to bake her mother a cake.

They started by gathering all of the supplies they needed.

"What do we need first, dad?" Lisa asked.

"Well, the recipe says that we need flour, sugar, cocoa, baking soda, and salt from the cupboard. Can you get those for us, kiddo?" Lisa's dad asked.

"Absolutely!" Lisa said.

Lisa went to the pantry, opened it up, and grabbed the flour from the bottom shelf, and the sugar, baking soda, and salt from the second shelf.

Then, she looked up and saw that the cocoa was all the way up on the top shelf.

"Can you grab it for me, please, dad?" Lisa asked.

"Great manners, Lisa! Of course, I can." her dad said, grabbing the cocoa off of the top shelf and putting it on the counter.

"What now, dad?" Lisa asked.

"Well, next, we need two eggs, buttermilk, butter, and vanilla." her dad answered.

"Great! I can do that!" Lisa said, opening the fridge to fetch the eggs, buttermilk, and butter.

"Where's the vanilla kept?" she asked, searching high and low for the vanilla.

"Whoops! That's in the cupboard!" her dad grinned, going back to the pantry to grab them the vanilla.

Lisa just giggled and grabbed a mixing bowl out of the cupboard.

"Is that everything?" Lisa asked.

"That is!" her dad smiled.

Lisa went back to the pantry, grabbed the footstool, and placed it by the counter where the mixing bowl was resting.

"Are we ready to get started?" she asked.

"We are! But first, we need the measuring cups and spoons! And a spatula." her dad said, pulling them out of the cupboard.

"Okay, let's get started!" he said.

"First, you need to measure out the flour. Can you measure out one and three-quarter cups of flour?" her dad asked, handing her the measuring cups.

"Absolutely!" Lisa said.

She carefully measured out the flour and dumped it into the mixing bowl.

"Great, now we need two cups of sugar. Can you put two cups of sugar into the bowl?" Lisa's dad asked.

"I sure can." Lisa grinned, adding two cups of sugar to the bowl.

"Now, we need three-quarters of a cup of cocoa powder."

"Okay!" Lisa smiled, adding the cocoa powder to the bowl.

"Can you add one and a half teaspoons of baking soda now, Lisa?" her dad asked, handing her the measuring spoons.

"Of course!" Lisa said, measuring out the baking soda and adding it to the bowl.

"Great, now we need three-quarters of a teaspoon of salt."

"Got it!" Lisa said, adding the salt.

As she added the salt, a little spilled over onto the counter.

"Oops!" Lisa said, looking up at her dad.

"No problem." he smiled, wiping it away with a damp cloth.

"Now what?" Lisa asked.

"Well, it says here that now you need to mix the dry ingredients together."

"Okay!" Lisa answered, using the spatula to mix the flour, sugar, cocoa powder, baking soda, and salt together.

The mixture darkened as the cocoa powder blended in with the other dry ingredients and started to look like the packaged cakes that her grandma sometimes purchased when she did not want to make a cake from scratch.

"Great, that looks good, Lisa. Now, let's add the wet ingredients together. Let's start with the eggs." her dad said, handing her two eggs.

"Can you do it by yourself?" he asked.

"I sure can!" Lisa smiled, carefully cracking the first egg over the side of the mixing bowl.

The side split and Lisa used her fingers to pry the egg open, revealing a gooey egg white and yolk inside.

She dumped the egg into the bowl, and then placed the eggshell to the side.

She cracked in the next egg, again prying the gooey egg open and letting the egg white and yolk slide into the bowl next to the other egg.

This time, she accidentally got some shell into the bowl.

"Oops! How do I get that out?" Lisa asked.

"Check this out," her dad said, taking half of the empty eggshell and scooping the broken piece out of the batter.

"Woah, how did you do that?" Lisa asked, amazed by how easily her dad pulled the eggshell out.

"Baker's secret." he winked.

"Okay, now let's add the buttermilk, we need one and a half cups of that."

Lisa's dad said, handing her the buttermilk.

Lisa measured out the milk and then poured it into the mixing bowl, watching the thick white milk mix together with the eggs on top of the dry ingredients.

"Done," Lisa said, putting the measuring cup down.

"Great, now let's add the butter. We need to melt it first, so I will do that." her dad said, measuring out half of a cup of butter and placing it in a small pot over medium heat, stirring it regularly to help it melt.

Once the butter was melted, Lisa's dad added it directly to the mixing bowl.

"Now, the vanilla. This is the last ingredient!" he said, handing her the vanilla.

"How much?" she asked.

"One tablespoon." he smiled, handing her the measuring spoons once again.

"Excellent." she grinned, pouring a tablespoon of vanilla into the mixing bowl.

"That's it! Mix it up!" Lisa's dad said.

As she started mixing the bowl, her dad turned on the stove and prepared the cake pans.

Meanwhile, Lisa used the spatula to mix together the ingredients in the bowl.

At first, it seemed like they were not coming together that well, but Lisa kept mixing and mixing.

Soon, all of the ingredients were coming together in a soupy wet mixture.

The batter was fairly wet and thick, but it looked like it would be absolutely delicious once it was done.

When Lisa was satisfied that she had mixed it all the way through, her dad gave it one last mix just to be sure that it was perfect.

Then, they poured the mixture into two separate cake pans, and her dad put them in the hot stove for her.

Lisa was so excited to finish these cakes for her mother that she stayed in the kitchen the whole time they were baking.

She sat on the floor in front of the oven, watching them rise.

At first, it looked like nothing was happening as the cakes simply sat in the oven baking.

Soon, however, the smell of chocolate cake began to fill the house, and the cakes slowly began to rise.

Lisa continued sitting there, watching the entire baking process play out before her very eyes as both of the cake rose and baked all the way through.

When the oven went off, Lisa stood back as her dad pulled the cakes out of the stove and poked a toothpick into the center of them to make sure they were baked all the way through.

"Perfection!" he smiled, showing her the toothpicks were completely clean upon coming out of the cake.

Exercise

Exercise to get a good night's sleep. If you exercise during the day, you will sleep better at night. Regular exercise can help you beat insomnia. In addition, it also helps you dwell in a deep sleep more.

- More vigorous exercise makes you sleep better at night. However, no matter how little they exercise, it will increase the quality of your sleep.

- It is essential to build a quality exercise habit. This is because you might not see the effect of regular exercise until after a couple of months.

Be Smart with Your Exercise Timing

There are many benefits of exercise, such as increased body temperature, boosting heart rate, and increasing the rate of metabolism. This is nice if you exercise in the morning or afternoon. Exercising in the evening, however, can be a recipe for disaster.

With this in mind, your vigorous exercise should end in the afternoon. If you must exercise in the evening, make it low impact and gentle like yoga, stretching, or walking.

Chapter 20. The Black Ball

During the early part of the morning, I was in a real rush trying to mop up the lobby, dusting the halls, replacing the old sand in the tall green jars with a new one, and clearing out the garbage which will later on in the day be taken to the incinerator for burning. I only got a short break to go get Mrs. Johnson a bottle of milk for her a new baby. She was always good for my boy. I had kicked off the day at 6 am, and at about 9 am, I had rushed hurriedly to our quarters at the garage, dressed my son and served him his breakfast, cereal, and fruits. He sat in his elevated seat rather thoughtful and stopped several times with his spoon just almost nearing his mouth, and then watched as I chewed on my toast bread.

"Son, what is the problem?

"Father, am I black?" Certainly not, you're brown. You definitely know that you're brown." Well, Jackie said yesterday that I was so black." "He was simply messing around with you. Don't allow them to joke around with you like that kid." "Father, being brown is much better than being black, isn't it?"(He was a young brown boy, four years of age, in his blue romper and when he laughed and talked around with is imaginary friends, you could detect the Black American ascent, in his gentle voice.) "Many individuals believed so. "I did say that American is superior to both son." Really dad?"I'm positive. Now, stop thinking about this insane talk of you being black, let me rush back and finish my chores, and daddy will be back to you when he's done."I left him with a picture book and toys to play with. He was such a lovely person, more than often, especially the quiet afternoons when I tried to read, he would come to me and anticipate a sweet treat or "picture movie," and also, I left him alone in the house most part of the days, as I attend to my assignments in the apartments.

I was already back to my post, brassing the front doors when I noticed there was a gentleman, who stood and watched me from the street. He was slender and red in his face, from the redness of the face, you could tell, he was one of those fellows who took those lengthy diets of specific foods. You see a lot of it from the profound south, and it's not unusual here from the southwest.

I could feel his piercing eyes on my back, as he just stood there, looking at me polishing the brass.

Berry, the boss, believed the value of my work is the luster of brass panels and door handles, therefore, I spent extra time working on the brass. It was almost his arrival time.

He would say, "Good morning, John," not looking at me, but at the brass.

"Good morning, sir," I'd say, all my attention at the brass instead of him.

There was always a reflection of him there. I've been there for him. I don't think he had any other real interest in life besides that brass, his cash, and his half-dozen or more plants in his office.

Everything should be perfect this morning. Whites were very specific and demanding in the precision of how work should be done. And as for that, two men were dismissed from the building across the street. I was not ready to lose my job over a man standing by the sidewalk, I had a son who required special foods, and I intended to enroll him to school coming term. Mainly, since my boss told one of my close acquaintance that he doesn't like that, "darned learned nigger." I vowed to dedicate my whole energy to my job. I ended up concentrating on the brass so much that I easily got spooked when the gentleman spoke. He said, "Howdy."

There was the anticipated drawl. But there was something lacking, generally something behind that drawl.

"Good morning." "Surely looks as if you're working fairly hard on that brass." "It gets fairly dirty all long night. They never leave that part out. You will always know when they had something to say to us. They become acquainted with us.

"How long have you been working here?" he inquired, with his elbow leaning against the column.

"Two months." Kept my back turned away from here as I went ahead doing my duty.

"Apart from you, are there any other black folks working here?" It is only me," I lied. In fact, there were two more brothers, just like me. That should be none of his concern, anyways.

"Do you have a lot to do?" I've got sufficient," I said. He should just go in and apply for this job; instead, I thought to myself. Why is this fellow disturbing me? Why provoke me to choke him? It seems like he doesn't know that we are not scared to fight his kind out of our way.

When I looked back to pick up more polish for my rag, I could see him remove a packet of cigarettes from his old blue coat pocket. The scarred hands were noticeable. They looked as if they were burnt.

"Have you ever smoked Durham?" he asked.

"Thank you, I don't smoke," I said.

He laughed.

"You are not used to such, isn't it?

"I am not used to what exactly? If I could hear anything more from this dude, there will be a blood bath.

"A person like me giving somebody like you something else apart from a rope." I put a hold on what I was doing, looking at him. With the packet in his extended open hand, he was standing there smiling. He had a lot of wrinkles around his eyes, and in exchange, I had to smile. Despite my spitefulness, I smiled back.

"Durham, you're not going to smoke, for real?"

I am sure, thanks," I said.

My smile deceived him. Nothing could change things between my kind and his, not even a smile."

"I know it ain't a lot," he said.

"This is hell a lot different." Once more, I paused, polishing the brass to see exactly the message he wanted to pass along.

"However, I have something of great value if your interested." he said, "Spill it," I said.

I thought he'd put one over the old "George" here. "You see, I'm coming out of a meeting with the union, and we're going to arrange all building service assistance in this district.

Perhaps, you have seen this in the papers?" I saw something about that, how does this really concern me?" Well, we're going to make them take some of this work away from you first. This will mean minimum working hours, increment in salaries, and a better working environment." "Wow, so what you really implying is that you will come here and kick me out."

Unions don't want representatives from the Black community.

"Are you implying certain unions don't. It was that way long ago, a lot of changed now." Listen here, gentleman, stop wasting your precious time and mine. Like anything else in the country, your goddamn unions are — for whites only. What led you to give a darn about Black man, anyway? Why do you want to coordinate with Black people?"His face turned a little white, at this moment.

"See these hands?" He extended his hands and spread them out."

"Yes," said I, staring at his turned face rather than his hands.

"Well, I got these scars in Alabama, Macon County, since I defended a black friend of mine of being in a different place on the day he had "allegedly" raped a woman. He was not guilty since, at the time of the occurrence of the event, I was with him. When it occurred— if it occurred, I and he had gone to borrow some seeds sixty miles away. These scars arose from the gasoline torch, and they barned me out of the county, in the name of "I am helping a black nigga, making the white woman sound like a liar. They lynched him to death, that very same night, and burnt his house down to ashes. Despite being sixty miles away, we were still executed for a need that we didn't commit."As he speaks, he kept looking at his outspread hands.

"Lord," was all I could utter out. I really felt awful when I got to have a close look at his hand for the first time. Indeed, it was hell for you. His skin was puckered and sapped, and it looked as if it had been in hot oil, well-fried hands.

"I have learned a lot since that moment," he said, "I have been at this sort of thing. It started with the Croppers, when they came to learn who I really was, they made it unbearable for me to live in the country, so I had to leave and come to town. It was first in Arkansas and here now.

And the more I'm moving, the more I see, the more I'm working. "Now his blue eyes, in his red skin, looked directly into my face. He looked very serious. I was quiet. I knew not what to tell him.

Maybe he was truthful and honest; I wasn't aware. Again, he smiled.

He said, "Listen." "At this moment, don't go and trying to figure all this out.

I would really love to see you at our meeting, with this kind of number, we are going to have numerous meetings starting tomorrow night. Tag any of your friends you wish." He gave me a card with a number and 8 p.m boldly written on it. You could see him smile when I took the card he and made it look as if he was shaking my hand and went down the street steps. As he walked away, I did notice that he limped.

Good morning, John, "said Mr. Berry. I turned, and there he was. He is wearing his Derby, lengthy black jacket, a stick, and those glasses that lay on the nose, and all. He stood there, looking into the brass like the evil and wicked Queen into her mirror, this is the kind of tales my boy enjoyed.

"Good morning, sir," I said.

I ought to have finished earlier.

Exercise

This CBT exercise can be especially helpful if you are dealing with depression. It works simply by creating a schedule of activities that you can look forward to, preferably in the near future. If you already have a journal, you can use it to write down your activities... This activity can be as simple as having coffee with a friend, playing a sport, or watching a movie. Keep in mind that the activity must be pleasant for you, but make sure that it is one that's not unhealthy. Aside from activities that you simply find pleasurable, you can also consider activities that can make you productive or give you a sense of mastery like learning a new skill. In many cases, doing something that makes you feel accomplished, no matter how small, can have a longer lasting effect.

Chapter 21. The Right Choice

This morning was like any other morning. I got up alone, got a cup of coffee alone, and sat by the window watching the sunrise... alone. If there was one thing, I thought about more than anything else; it is that I was tired of being alone. I went grocery shopping, and what did I see? Men and women together. When I went to the park, what did I see, young men and young women together? Even just walking down the street, I see couples. I was getting older and did not want to get really old and just fade away by myself. We are meant to be with each other, so that doesn't happen so that when one of us gets sick, the other one can take care of us and love us. I was so certain I was right about this. I knew that just because I had this huge fixation on watching other couples, it didn't mean that there were no other people alone and lonely like me, but that's how it felt, and I was just tired of it.

My name is Johnathon Smith, and I live in the windy city. Chicago has always been my home. I was born here, and I got my first job here when I was 15 years old. Today I am a ghostwriter for a large firm right in the center of downtown in a big high-rise building, but I work from home. I write books. I only go into the office when they have mandatory meetings, and these days that is a rare occasion. This means I don't even need to leave the house other than for groceries and the occasional walk.

"How do people get together? How do they do it?" I asked myself. "Do the stars have to be just right or what?" I mumbled to myself. It was Monday morning, and I had just had my coffee. I went into the bathroom to look at myself. "I'm not a bad looking guy!" I told myself. "I should be able to get a woman to love me, shouldn't I?" I questioned. It was 2018, and everyone had access to the Internet. Well, I guess nearly everyone. "I should get back on those dating sites," I mused. At least it's something, and you never know. Maybe this time I'll get lucky.

I had tried that before, and it was a disaster. Every woman I liked didn't like me. Every woman who contacted me, I didn't like for some reason. Usually, it was just a feeling. I understand my emotions and my sense of chemistry and can always clearly know if a woman gives me that "Woo-Hood" feeling or not. I have met those who do not give me that feeling before, thinking well maybe I'm just wrong about this chemistry thing. I'm not. It was worse in person than looking at their picture, so I swore never to do that again. What a pain to meet somebody for coffee and know the minute you lay eyes on her that she is not "the one" and then have to suffer sitting with her for an hour before squirming out of it with some lame excuse. That's just embarrassing and stupid. That's all it is, and I won't do it again. For that matter, this whole Internet Dating thing is stupid. Forget that; there has to be a better way to meet a woman naturally.

The months passed by, and nothing changed. Work, work, and more work and don't get me wrong, I love my job, and I have always loved to write, but I was just very bored with everything else in my life. Then one morning, I was finishing up a book for the firm, and like always, I immediately went to our worksite and looked for another one to begin work on. I did this all the time. Finish one book and right away without taking a breath, go find another one to start. "Maybe that's the problem." I thought to myself. "Maybe I need to take a breather between work assignments and go out; live a little." I wondered.

"Oh well," I thought, "At least I have my health and my job. I do love my job."

When I got to the worksite, I browsed through all the topics and started to get bored. I wasn't finding anything I liked. I was just about to give up on today's list when I saw something that jumped out at me. It was a title. "Meditation and Mindfulness for Beginners." "I could do that one," I said to myself. See, that's the thing about writing. When you write about a topic that you don't know much about, by the time you get done, you know a great deal about it. "Maybe this one will change my life." I pondered. I selected the topic and got right to work on it.

By that evening, I was quite getting excited. I began to think about trying this meditation thing out for myself. What would I have to lose? I wrote and wrote, and I understood what I was writing. "Well, that doesn't always happen now, does it?" I asked myself. When I got to a break-off point, I stopped and took a short break.

I went into my bedroom and put some cushions on the floor and then sat down in the position the instructions said to sit. I listened to my breath and became relaxed in its rhythm. I started to fall asleep, and my mind said, "Hey, we're tired. Why are you sitting up? Take us to bed so we can rest!" I recalled the instructions said this would happen and to just ignore it, so that's what I did. Then I felt the eye of my mind coming out. It was strange at first, but, like my breathing, I got a sort of rhythm going and stayed with it. Very soon, something wonderful happened. I began to hear voices. They weren't my voice but another deeper voice. It said, "Everybody has a task!" and then I just thought about what I had just heard and wondered if I had heard it at all. But clearly, I had.

I stayed with it and started to feel really good. I mean really well and I loved it. I felt as though I was nearly floating up off the floor. I was flying, and it was just me. I was doing it all by myself. Then I thought, "If this is real, I will know it when I stop." And right then, I opened my eyes and looked around. I felt better than I have felt in a long time.

I wanted to learn more, so I went back to work on the book. I remembered that I had read a word. Something with the word mind. Mind something. Then I found it. The word was mindfulness, and it goes together with meditation. I went to a search engine and looked it up. "Mindfulness," there it was. It said that it was an awareness of one's own feelings, surroundings, and sensations. Being in the moment. Be here now. I liked it, and I told myself that this just might be what is holding me back in the dating world. "I will be mindful, and I will meditate, and then we'll see." I thought.

The next morning, I went down to my local coffee shop and got a table in the back. I brought my laptop and hooked it up to power and then went up to the counter to order my coffee. "May I help you?" the little lady behind the counter said. "Ah, yes, I'll have a hot Latte with a touch of chocolate, please," I told her. "Oh, that's my favorite too." She told me with a big smile. I looked at her again, she had pretty eyes, and she was just standing there staring at me. "Okay," she finally said. "One hot Latte coming right up!" I paid her and went back to my seat.

Something was different. I was getting much more attention from the people around me, and I had a pretty good idea why. I was being mindful, which made me more relaxed, which was an attractive quality that people really liked. Then, some people started filling in the tables around me. Very soon, there were only a couple of seats left, and they were at my table, and a very cute lady walked in all alone. "Hmmmm," I thought to myself. "I wonder if she'll take her coffee to go." I watched her with great interest, and then she suddenly turned and walked straight towards me. "Hello," she said to me. "You don't mind some company, do you?" Noticing that she had her hands full, I jumped up and pulled her chair out for her. "Why thank you, kind sir," she said. "What a lovely voice," I thought. I sat back down and pretended to be busy doing something on my computer.

"What are you working on?" she asked me. She was interested in me. She was honestly interested. I shut my computer and said, "I'm a writer." "Oh, really?" she responded. "You must tell me about your work sometime." She said with a sultry tone. "Sometime?" I thought to myself. "That means another time, which means she wants to see me again or even maybe do something together right now!" My thoughts were all a swirl, and then I realized it and hoped she hadn't noticed. She hadn't. She was fishing in her purse for something. "What's your name?" she asked me. "My— Uh—Oh, Johnathon," I said. "I'm Christie." She told me. And before long we were like old friends. We talked about what she does and what she wants out of life. Then we talked about what I want out of my life, and it seemed that we both thought the same thing. "Can I buy you lunch?" I blurted. "Oh, I don't think they serve lunch here," Christie said to me. "No, I mean, can we go to lunch together someplace else. That is, would you like to join me for lunch?"

"I would love that Johnathon. I love your name, by the way – Johnathon." She said to me with a smile. Since we were in the city, there were restaurants everywhere, so we just walked down the sidewalk for a couple of blocks, found a place we liked, and went in and had lunch. I knew from the time we met that if all went well, she might be the woman for whom I had been waiting. So far, so good. After lunch, she gave me her number, and we stayed in touch. out!"

Exercise

This is one example of what exposure therapy is. It may sound complicated, but it's actually very simple. It works with you listing down situations you would normally avoid. If you have social anxiety, for instance, you may typically avoid greeting another person first. List down at least ten similar situations and rate each of them on how distressed or anxious you think you would be if you engaged in such activity. Rate each from 0 to 10. Doing this exercise will help you identify situations you find difficult or challenging the most, as well as help you decide which situations to address first and in what order.

Chapter 22. The Pokémon Monster

The heat was sweltering on the road surface, vibrations rising from the asphalt.

Sven looked up from his cell phone and watched the air vibrate before his eyes.

Hm, that is not the case, he thought.

He was not yet used to roaming outside.

From his 7th birthday, he had received a computer from his parents, and he had spent years of his life behind that thing.

He was able to play like the best, so he played this game every day for hours.

This meant that he would not have been outside for years.

But in the meantime, thanks to the new Pokémon game, he came out daily and even for many hours. Even his arms tanned for the first time since his younger years.

Sven was now 23 years old.

He felt comfortable the way it was now.

Sven was a tall skinny boy with a backpack on his back, simple, average clothing, his hair was long and wild, and he wore a dark frame on his nose.

He was not interested in fashion, he was not so interested in it, and in fact, he still wore the same kind of clothing as when he was seven years old.

But in the meantime, he saw something of the world again, the living, the people, and somewhere he realized what he had missed all those years.

He saw people again; he even spoke to people. That wasn't easy; his voice seemed to be stuck because he had not spoken to anyone for years.

But now he learned to communicate again, and he liked that.

Today it was bizarre hot, 35 degrees even.

But he still wanted to score a new Pokémon.

He had been around for many hours, from the park to the hospital and back because somewhere hidden among the trees, there had to be a Pokémon.

It was quite busy, despite the heat.

Sven squeezed his eyes together for a moment to focus on his smartphone screen; he went ahead again. He peered at the image and saw nothing.

For months he had studied this. He played Pokémon daily.

He dreamed on the night of Pokémon's that were everywhere, everywhere around humanity in the strangest places.

A virtual world that seemed to merge more and more with reality.

Now, after all these years of gaming, Sven didn't know much about reality anymore.

It was a beautiful summer evening that night, and Sven walked with his bowl of fries to a park bench.

There were two more people on the bench, also looking for the Pokémon nearby.

They agreed to continue in the dark with each other.

Hunting for the Pokémon in the forest.

Somewhere there had to be one.

Around midnight they were still walking among the bushes.

It was, fortunately, full moon, so they could still see where they were walking.

Sven, however, stumbled over a tree stump and lay flat on the ground for a moment.

By the time he got up, he no longer saw his two fellow seekers.

They suddenly disappeared. He still called them, but strangely enough, they didn't hear him or were too far away.

Sven shrugged and walked on.

He is continuously staring at his mobile.

Somewhere farther away, he saw a strange red light shining on his screen.

So, he had to be there.

Sven walked quickly towards the light.

He looked through his screen at the Pokémon he would see first!

Yes, there was something to see, but what was it?

Sven's breath caught him in his throat.

A devil being stared at him on his screen.

Sven looked up from his cell phone and saw nothing.

He only saw the darkness of the trees. He looked at his screen again and saw another monstrous creature staring at him.

Sven suddenly became intensely dizzy. He rubbed his forehead once, which was damp; was it sweat, or was it blood?

In the moonlit darkness, Sven was shocked to see a black spot on his hand, so blood?

He felt his forehead again, a big cut, nothing serious, right? Had he been unconscious for a moment?

Had his fellow seekers left without him?

Sven didn't know, but for him was an ugly creature who would represent a Pokémon.

He peered at the screen again, yes, look there it was. Still, the creature had come closer.

Sven was shocked again because it was a filthy creature, despicably ugly and creepy.

This was not what he knew as a Pokémon ... how they could put it like a Pokémon creature in a forest.

Sven didn't understand.

He was aiming for the creature for him.

The honor was his, didn't he? The red mist around the creature grew bigger...

A strange rotting scent passed by him; Sven did not dare to look up from his smartphone.

Oh my god, he thought.

Something gasped in his neck, a stinking warm breath.

He felt claws clasped on his shoulders, with big nails, stinging painfully into his skin.

Sven wanted to turn around, but that didn't work, paralyzed with fear, and the hands stopped him because they were reliable.

Who are you? What do you want from me...? Sven stammered...

I, I am the Pokémon monster!

The monster hissed behind him; you are the first to see one.

You have found almost all Pokémon's, and there is a reward in return.

Me! The Satanic Pokémon Monster and you were the first to find me.

What a miracle and how long this took, the creature laughed in his neck.

And now? Sven asked the Pokémon monster.

The monster laughed hard in his ears, and Sven felt the claws go toward his back.

Sven broke out in a sweat, what was going to happen, and how could this happen? This was not the game as he knew it.

What do you want from me, Poke monster?

Oh that, the monster muttered hot, leave that to me, boy.

Those who find me can, of course, pay for it, after this, you will be the king of the Pokémon's!

I am the finish line of the game, you see.

Sven felt the claws move toward his belt and deftly buckled the belt.

What will you do with me...? Screamed Sven in a high voice.

Hahahahaa the Pokémon monster laughed, what am I going to do?

You will notice that.

The Pokémon monster skillfully slipped down Sven's pants.

There Sven stood in his bare ass in the middle of the night in the forest, who would find him, he thought anxiously.

With enormous power, the Pokémon monster pushed Sven forward on his knees.

Oh god, neeeeeeeee…. Sven exclaimed. Neeeeeeeeee not that!! ?? The Pokémon monster once sniffed violently.

Hmmmmmm, the monster exclaimed.

Unfortunately, from behind a large sex organ boiling in Sven's anus.

Sven screamed in pain and lost consciousness.

The sun was already rising, and Sven was still unconscious on the ground in the grass with his smartphone clutched in his fingers.

The two fellow seekers finally saw him and were relieved.

Sven!

Sven woke up, one of them called.

Sven opened his eyes; his anus hurt a lot; that was all he felt. Oh, he moaned, oh, what a pain.

He told what had happened to him.

The fellow seekers looked at him with compassion. What a *** dude, hahaha, you must have been raped here by a gay man!

No, serious, Sven exclaimed in despair, look here on my mobile.

He showed the photo, I am now the king of Pokémon monsters, he muttered almost crying.

Stunned, the fellow seekers looked at the photo of a horrible devil monster.

It grinned at them from the smartphone.

My god and that raped you last night in this forest?

I stop this game hear one of the fellow seekers said if all this awaits us.

I also said the other; I don't have to.

No, he said Sven with a vague smile on his face, the pain almost hit him.

Nobody wants this!

The fellow seekers dragged Sven home, stumbling through the park, tears running down his cheeks.

At the hospital, they decided to have Sven examined; he was allowed to stay for a few days immediately because of a torn entourage entrance.

The fellow seekers were Sven's best friends, but they never played Pokémon again.

The game soon ended when the stories circulated that some people couldn't believe.

Yet there were more stories all over the world about that Poke monster; it seemed to be a creature that had been summoned from the dark worlds thanks to CERN.

They did not know how to get rid of it, because they could never get hold of it, but he did get hold of people, and considerably.

Often in a dark forest. dance.

Exercise

This is another type of exposure therapy, but this time, it involves you thinking about a memory that produced very strong negative feelings within you and analyzing that situation. If you've have fight recently with a close kin, for instance, and they said something that hurt you, you can think of that situation and try to remember every detail of the scenario. Once you've had a good memory of the event, you then try to label the thoughts and emotions you've had during that event and try to remember the urges that you felt at the time. Did you think of running away from the situation? Did you think of crying, or maybe yelling at the other person?

Visualizing such negative situation for extended periods can help you eliminate that memory's ability to trigger you and reduce the chances of you avoiding it. The reason is that exposing yourself to the urges you felt in the situation and surviving the memory takes away the power of that particular memory.

Chapter 23. New Orleans

In some cities, the history of it is just something tourists come to see for a few days, but in New Orleans, history is part of everyday life, and the locals live in it full time. A still functioning piece of history is used every day to bring people about their lives and have done so for a hundred years. The one thing that lives up to this the most is the streetcars of New Orleans. In most cities, artifacts like streetcars are something the locals avoid. Stepping on a tram in New Orleans, you are as likely to sit beside a local musician as you would be to sit beside a tourist here to see some musicians play while in town.

For my trip through the many diverse neighborhoods of Nola, I start on the St. Charles line, the oldest running continuous streetcar in the world. For over 150 years, this olive-green streetcar has been rumbling through these streets. Taking people to and from work, play, and everything in between. The route forms a crescent through the Central Business District along Canal Street and into the prestigious Uptown neighborhood. I pay my fair of 1.25 in exact change as requested by the sign on the front of the car and take a window seat a few rows behind the operator. Inside, the seats are the original mahogany benches, and the brass fittings have stood the test of time. The operator uses a lever system to control the small wheels that the roomy streetcar is perched on. With the twist of their wrist, the car lurches into action. These were not built for aerodynamics or comfort. Still, the old-fashioned charm of the hundred-year-old public transportation quickly grows on me.

The car rocks side to side as it picks up speed toward the next station, and as it lumbers through the city, passengers hop on and off at the different stations. The track takes a sweeping turn at the curve of the crescent, and the driver effortlessly directs the large metal box on wheels around the bend and down the legendary St. Charles Avenue. Soon we're in the historic Uptown section of New Orleans. Here along the east bank of the mighty Mississippi river, we chug along the track through a long tunnel of oak tree branches. The trunks rooted in front yards of stately mansions that line parts of the street. The houses are from picture books and movies, emphasizing the charm and romance of Nola. Beautifully keep estates, with large front porches that sweep all the way around the side of the white or yellow home, with ornate columns that hold up the second-floor balcony.

The streetcar rocks its way through the old neighborhood picking up and dropping off locals and tourists alike. Near the end of the line, I jump off at a station across from a large white cathedral. It has arched doorways, spires on every peak, and a bell tower that reaches high above the leafy oak tree canopy. A few blocks down a few side streets, lined with more homes each with a unique charm but all within the same style of porches, columns, and balconies, there is a small cemetery with a large population, the Lafayette cemetery takes up only one city block but with its many family mausoleums is the final home of family members stretching back as far as the city's history does. The large stone structures, each with their own unique charm, remind me of the rows of stately homes I just passed on the streetcar and how we all want a little piece of beauty with us no matter where we are in life.

I wander the narrow paths noting how ferns grow from the cracks that have developed over time. Indicating that life will always find a way to spring forth from even the smallest of opportunities. The space has a somber effect, but the splashes of green reminds me that there is always hope and something to believe in. If these ferns can thrive here, in the forgotten cracks of history in New Orleans, then I imagine that any struggle I face is manageable if just persevere.

Leaving the cemetery, I hear a lively jazz band striking up, and I find my way to the bar they are playing in. The band is on a stage inside with a few people scattered about the room listening in, music is everywhere in this city, and I think it needs to be. Like the ferns in the cracks, New Orleans relies on the little glimmers of life. The streetcar still running after all these years. The old homes with porches that housed many families and played host to their triumphs and struggles. The jazz standards passed down from generation to generation. All of these have stood the test of time and wear layers of history like strands of beads around the necks of mardi grass participants, one-part beauty, and one-part a weighty ache. I enter the bar and find a stool near the street to watch the band and the streetcar, both chugging forward with a rhythm that is uniquely New Orleans.

Exercise

Steps for increasing effectiveness of the story:

1. What do you want to achieve from reading this?

2. Think about one thing you have achieved today.

3. Say to yourself "When I read this story then..."

Chapter 24. The Bell of Atri

Atri is the name of a little town in Italy. It is a very old town, and is built half-way up the side of a steep hill.

A long time ago, the King of Atri bought a fine large bell, and had it hung up in a tower in the market place. A long rope that reached almost to the ground was fastened to the bell. The smallest child could ring the bell by pulling upon this rope. "It is the bell of justice," said the king.

When at last everything was ready, the people of Atri had a great holiday. All the men and women and children came down to the market place to look at the bell of justice. It was a very pretty bell, and was, polished until it looked almost as bright and yellow as the sun.

"How we should like to hear it ring!" they said. Then the king came down the street.

"Perhaps he will ring it," said the people; and everybody stood very still, and waited to see what he would do.

But he did not ring the bell. He did not even take the rope in his hands. When he came to the foot of the tower, he stopped, and raised his hand.

"My people," he said, "do you see this beautiful bell? It is your bell; but it must never be rung except in case of need. If any one of you is wronged at any time, he may come and ring the bell; and then the judges shall come together at once, and hear his case, and give him justice. Rich and poor, old and young, all alike may come; but no one must touch the rope unless he knows that he has been wronged."

Many years passed by after this. Many times did the bell in the market place ring out to call the judges together. Many wrongs were righted, many ill-doers were punished. At last the hempen rope was almost worn out. The lower part of it was untwisted; some of the strands were broken; it became so short that only a tall man could reach it.

"This will never do," said the judges one day. "What if a child should be wronged? It could not ring the bell to let us know it."

They gave orders that a new rope should be put upon the bell at once,--a rope that should hang down to the ground, so that the smallest child could reach it. But there was not a rope to be found in all Atri. They would have to send across the mountains for one, and it would be many days before it could be brought. What if some great wrong should be done before it came? How could the judges know about it, if the injured one could not reach the old rope?

"Let me fix it for you," said a man who stood by. He ran into his garden, which was not far away, and soon came back with a long grapevine in his hands. "This will do for a rope," he said; and he climbed up, and fastened it to the bell. The slender vine, with its leaves and tendrils still upon it, trailed to the ground.

"Yes," said the judges, "it is a very good rope. Let it be as it is."

Now, on the hill-side above the village, there lived a man who had once been a brave knight. In his youth he had ridden through many lands, and he had fought in many a battle. His best friend through all that time had been his horse,--a strong, noble steed that had borne him safe through many a danger. But the knight, when he grew older, cared no more to ride into battle; he cared no more to do brave deeds; he thought of nothing but gold; he became a miser. At last he sold all that he had, except his horse, and went to live in a little hut on the hill-side. Day after day he sat among his money bags, and planned how he might get more gold; and day after day his horse stood in his bare stall, half-starved, and shivering with cold.

"What is the use of keeping that lazy steed?" said the miser to himself one morning. "Every week it costs me more to keep him than he is worth. I might sell him; but there is not a man that wants him. I cannot even give him away. I will turn him out to shift for himself, and pick grass by the roadside. If he starves to death, so much the better."

So the brave old horse was turned out to find what he could among the rocks on the barren hill-side. Lame and sick, he strolled along the dusty roads, glad to find a blade of grass or a thistle. The boys threw stones at him, the dogs barked at him, and in all the world there was no one to pity him.

One hot afternoon, when no one was upon the street, the horse chanced to wander into the market place. Not a man nor child was there, for the heat of the sun had driven them all indoors. The gates were wide open; the poor beast could roam where he pleased. He saw the grapevine rope that hung from the bell of justice. The leaves and tendrils upon it were still fresh and green, for it had not been there long. What a fine dinner they would be for a starving horse!

He stretched his thin neck, and took one of the tempting morsels in his mouth. It was hard to break it from the vine. He pulled at it, and the great bell above him began to ring. All the people in Atri heard it. It seemed to say,--

"Some one has done me wrong!
Some one has done me wrong!
Oh! come and judge my case!
Oh! come and judge my case!
For I've been wronged!"

The judges heard it. They put on their robes, and went out through the hot streets to the market place. They wondered who it could be who would ring the bell at such a time. When they passed through the gate, they saw the old horse nibbling at the vine.

"Ha!" cried one, "it is the miser's steed. He has come to call for justice; for his master, as everybody knows, has treated him most shamefully."

"He pleads his cause as well as any dumb brute can," said another."And he shall have justice!" said the third.

Meanwhile a crowd of men and women and children had come into the market place, eager to learn what cause the judges were about to try.

When they saw the horse, all stood still in wonder. Then every one was ready to tell how they had seen him wandering on the hills, unfed, uncared for, while his master sat at home counting his bags of gold.

"Go bring the miser before us," said the judges. And when he came, they bade him stand and hear their judgment.

"This horse has served you well for many a year," they said. "He has saved you from many a peril. He has helped you gain your wealth.

Therefore we order that one half of all your gold shall be set aside to buy him shelter and food, a green pasture where he may graze, and a warm stall to comfort him in his old age."

The miser hung his head, and grieved to lose his gold; but the people shouted with joy, and the horse was led away to his new stall and a dinner such as he had not had in many a day.

Exercise

Identifying stress

Have your child consider the prompts below. You can provide them with the examples so they can better understand how they can identify their own emotions in specific situations and pick up on the cues their body gives. Then brainstorm activities your child can do to help them feel better when they are experiencing these emotions.

I feel stressed when...
- There is too much noise.
- My parents fight.
- I forget something for school.
- I don't know the answer to something.
- I am asked to do too many things.
- I can't remember what I am supposed to be doing.
- I can't find anything I need.

When I feel stressed by body feels...
- Shaky
- My head hurts
- My body feels tired
- My heart feels like it is racing

When I am stressed I can...

- Ask for help
- Take a deep breath and count to five
- Read a book
- Listen to calming music
- Go for a walk
- Color

I FEEL STRESSED WHEN:
_____
_____
_____
_____

WHEN I FEEL STRESSED MY BODY:
_____
_____
_____
_____

WHEN I FEEL STRESSED I CAN:
_____
_____
_____
_____

Chapter 25. The Mermaid

It was a beautiful evening. As I stood by the ocean, the cool breeze from the sea hit my completely, making me smile in contentment. I could get used to this.

As I looked forward, I noticed the sun was getting closer to setting, with the sky looking a beautiful orange with a subtle amount of pink.

I smiled to myself. It was the perfect moment. I never wanted this moment to go away. I did have to head back soon though, because I felt like...if I stayed out here for too long, I'd probably get lost in the dark or something.

Still, the quiet nature of the sea as it hit the sand, the feel of the soft, white sand beneath my toes, and the cool sea breeze that had a briny taste in the air made me feel good and happy. I felt whole, I felt amazing, and I felt like...I could never get rid of that feeling. Life felt good, and I didn't think about the worries that were in my life.

Then, I heard it.

The splash.

I turned, unable to find anything around. I heard it once more, arousing my curiosity.

"Who's there?" I asked, turning to my left, and then over to the right. There was nothing.

Then what was that sound coming from?

I heard the sound of a thud. It was near the rock that was to my right. I went over there, wading in the water, checking to see what it was.

The sight in front of me threw me off.

It was the most beautiful mermaid I'd ever seen. I thought that they were fictional. But here I was, looking at the most beautiful creature I'd ever seen.

She wore two meager shells, had a large, purple-green tail, and soft, brown hair that cascaded down into tendrils. As I looked at this beautiful form, I felt like I was being tested.

Should I check on her? Was it the right thing to do? I honestly didn't even know anymore, and I felt like there was so much more going on here. I felt like... with everything that was happening maybe there was something deeper here. But she was quite beautiful, and she didn't seem to be awake. I grabbed her, hoisting her into my arms. She was much lighter than I thought she would be. Shortly after, I brought her over to the edge of the beach, keeping her in the water, but out of the depths. I was glad to do that too, because if she stayed there, I think she might've drowned.

She was still unconscious for a little while. I checked her vitals, to see if there was any sign of life. So far, she was somewhat alive. She had a heart, but her breathing was strange. It was not like a human's.

I started to freak out. What do I do about this? How do I...fix this? I looked at her, trying to figure out what it was that I wanted to do. After a bit, I noticed her eyes begin to open up. She looked at me with the most beautiful greenish-blue eyes, her mouth agape.

"What are you doing?" she said, scrambling over to the water.

"You almost hit your head. I wanted to make sure that you were okay," I told her.

She looked at me about to say something about my actions, but then, she stopped.

"I see. Thank you. I... I got hit by a boat, and I was rendered unconscious. I guess my tail tried to get me to a safe area. I don't really remember what happened, but my head is killing me," she said.

I nodded, understanding her pain.

"I get that. Do you want me to check your head? I'm a doctor, you know," I said.

"That would be nice. I heard of those types of people on the surface, but I never met one until now," she said.

I looked at her body, to see if there were any other marks or bruises, but there was nothing. I checked her head, and luckily, she seemed fine so far.

She was safe, but I had many different questions to ask her. She looked at me with a look of curiosity, and then, I shook my head.

"You're fine. But that was quite a hit you took. Are you sure you're okay?" I asked.

"Yeah. My parents told me not to talk to humans, and I'm not comfortable with humans. I haven't been, at least since I was a child. But you...you seem different. You're nice," she said.

I blushed.

"Thank you. I haven't done anything super amazing or anything. I was just a doctor, heading back home after a relaxing day, and I wanted to make sure you were kept safe," I told her.

"Well thanks. By the way, are you free tomorrow?" she asked.

What did she want to do tomorrow? Did she want to meet up here? I mean, I wouldn't mind that. I haven't been on a date in a long time, let alone with someone so beautiful. I didn't think I would get this lucky, but here we are.

"I mean yeah. After work of course. That'll be around noon though, since I work first shift. Why?"

"I wouldn't mind spending time with you. As a way to thank you for what you did. If you're fine with that," she said.

I blushed. I mean, did this mermaid really want to spend time with me? I was curious about her, but I had no idea what she had planned.

"Sure. I mean, what's the plan anyways?"

"You'll see. Just wear something you don't mind getting wet," she said.

I nodded, grinning towards her.

"By the way, what's your name?"

"Althea. And you?"

I told her my name, and her expression softened.

"Well, you're the first human to make me feel happy, to make me realize, there is a chance I can trust someone like you. So, thanks. I guess I'll be seeing you tomorrow," she said.

I nodded.

"Will do Althea."

I went back, and I wrote down my experience. I would journal my entire experience with the mysterious Althea, and I was curious about how this would go.

The two of us connected I felt. It was the first time in a very long time I actually felt a connection with someone. Most girls were just interested in a professional relationship and nothing more. I felt happy knowing this strange creature wanted to see me. Even though it might not matter at the end of the day, I felt it was worthwhile.

For the rest of the night, I slept, dreaming of the fun and excitement that I would have. During work, it went as it normally did. I worked at a hospital as their nurse practitioner, but I worked the early shift. Mostly because it would let me have a full day to do other things.

And of course, today would be a fun day.

I went to the beach around the time that I said I would, and when I did, I noticed she was already there. She waited near the rock, looking at me with a smile on her face. I then noticed that there was a smirk she had on her face.

"There you are. I was wondering if you'd show up," she teased.

"I had a plan to do so," I told her. She smiled at me, but then handed me a small phial.

"I wanted to give this to you once we were together again. Take a sip of it," she said.

I did so, and that's when I noticed the changes in my body. Instead of legs, I had a tail. I gasped, holding onto the rock for support.

"W-what did you do?" I asked.

"Relax silly. It's just a potion. It only works for 12 hours, but it lets you be a mermaid. I figured we could...swim around together," she explained.

I blushed. I didn't expect her to do this. I quickly nodded, getting my bearings as I clung to the rock.

"You don't have to worry or anything. Just take it easy," she said with a smile.

"Alright," I replied.

I closed my eyes, focused my breathing, and soon, I relaxed. I started to realize over time that I was actually able to swim easily. Together, we both went into the water. I kept my head above water, but then, Althea smiled.

"Don't worry, you can breathe in the water. I have gills up my sides," she said, showing me the small little pouches of air. I looked at my body, and sure enough I did too. I trusted her, and soon, the two of us went into the water.

At first, I freaked out. I thought that I had to breathe. But then, I realized I didn't need to, and because of that, I was able to swim quite easily. Swimming involved moving the tail in certain ways. Althea showed me, holding onto me as I awkwardly flopped about.

I then figured how to control it. It took me a few tries, but then, I was swimming around. It was freeing, and when I looked in the water, I saw all the animals clearly.

There were schools of fish, and a whole cluster of coral and even a few sea anemones here. Althea smiled, excited to see that I enjoyed this.

"Is it okay for me to follow you to your home?" I asked.

"Yeah. I told my dad about you. He said it's weird that I like a human so much, but I told him that you saved my life ad we take pride in that sort of thing here," she replied.

That explained it. I mean, I was going to stick around anyways. I followed her to the little pathway that was to the right, following it about until I finally got to; the small little city that I saw.

It really did look like something out of a Disney movie. There were a bunch of mermaids swimming around, a few of them with dolphins and other creatures. I noticed the large, expansive coral buildings, and every time I swam by one, I noticed all the little plants and animals.

Exercise

Sometimes it's easier to identify values based on what we like to do. For example, I might realize based on activities I've listed that meeting new people is important to me. Identifying that value can then help me brainstorm other ways of meeting new people.

Our values can help us come up with activities that support them, and activities we find rewarding can clue us in to what we value.

VALUES & ACTIVITIES FORM

RELATIONSHIPS

Value: --

Activity: ---

Activity: ---

Activity: ---

Value: --

Chapter 26. Finding Shorty

The summer has broken out in the small village of Sawbuck. Libby and her friends have long been waiting for the big heat wave to finally be able to bathe again at the Lasse quarry. Already in the morning the air smells of summer. Libby is on his way to Popped to pick him up at school. Alex is coming too. At the corner of the Gaushala Libby makes as usual a larger arc around the house of the old Belbin. Old Belbin has been living there for ages. At least he looks like this. Somehow the old man has something scary with all the wrinkles on his face and bony hands.

Libby and her friends once danced on Belbin's property. Of course, he caught her. Old Belbin just gets it all. As if he had his eyes and ears everywhere. He chased the children from his property with his cane in hand. Since then, they have avoided the house.

Libby is driving past the house. Usually it is the same picture every morning. The old Belbin stands on his lawn bleating and complaining to the neighbor, because his dog has allegedly done his business there again. The neighbor does not answer anymore. He takes his daughter to the car and pretends he does not hear Belbin. That makes old Belbin so mad that he gets louder.

The three friends have also seen how the old Belbin complained loudly to his neighbor, because the dog had barked all night. He barely had an eye - heard the old man yelling. Whereby the dog of the Knaggs really likes to bark at night. At least that's what Libby's mom says. She often protects old Belbin and always tells how friendly he used to be when Mrs. Belbin was still alive.

But today, nothing is to be seen or heard of old Belbin. Also Mr. Knaggs is not - as usual - in the driveway. Libby stops for a moment and scratches his head thoughtfully. "That's funny," she thinks. "Did something happen to old Belbin?" She would like to check. But he does not dare and then he continues.

After a few minutes, Libby arrives at Popped. Of course, Popped is not his real name. Actually, his name is Holger. But because he is a bit more stable, it looks kind of funny when he runs. At some point, Alex said: "Look, Holger comes running hoppeldipoppel." Alex and Libby had to laugh so hard that they called Holger from then only Popped. By now he's so used to hearing Holger.

Alex is coming too. "Hey Alex - almost at the same time - what?" Libby shouts to Alex. Alex grins: "Oh, Libby, did not even see you - yes, funny." Then the front door flies open and popped trumpets: "Well send her thick - everything in step?" That's Popper's typical way. Always the big mouth in front path.

Libby shakes his head: "I think you'll never change Popped!" Popped beams over his ears: "But never my dear Libby - you sweetie!" He says and shakes Libby's hand. Libby has to laugh. But then she gets serious: "Hey guys, you know what I've been watching today? Old Belbin was not complaining. "Popped is closing his bike lock:" Oh, well, did he swallow himself or what? "Libby shakes his head:" No, seriously. He was not there. And Knaggs was not in the driveway. I was thinking about looking to see if something had happened to the old Belbin. "

Alex thinks: "Funny it is." But Popped interferes immediately: "Nah no people, you can forget that right away. You probably do not remember how the old Zeisel chased us off the grounds with a fat club.

You can eat that nice. The thick one always gets it first! I cannot get ten more horses! "Libby rolls her eyes:" Oh Popped, you always have to overdo everything! That was a walking stick and not a club! "

Popped waves down: "I do not care what you tell Libby. In my story that was a fat stick and I'll stick with it. "Alex shakes his head but then says," Either way, popped is right Libby. That brings nothing but trouble. In addition, we are slowly getting late. We should really go to school. If I'm late again, my dad turns right on the bike. "Libby nods and the three go.

The school day passes quickly and Libby does not mention the topic with the old Belbin anymore. In the afternoon, the three friends drive to the Lasse quarry to test the water for temperature. Libby keeps his foot in the water and immediately winced. "Burr, is that still cold! The lake has probably not noticed the summer is. "Alex and Popped laugh. Then Alex says, "We'll keep those few days off now. In addition, soon holidays. "Popped nods:" Right! I am already counting the days. We have another week until the summer holidays. Then it will finally be donated again! Stop schoolwork and stuff! "

The next morning Libby drives her track as usual to pick up Popped. But there is no sign of old Belbin. Shortly before Popper's house she sees Mr. Knaggs, who is putting a leaflet on the fence. Libby stops to look at it. On the leaflet is a missing message for the dog of the Knaggs. "That makes sense," she thinks. "If the King's dog ran away, then old Belbin has no reason to complain."

Mr. Knaggs sees Libby and approaches: "Hello Libby, Shorty disappeared the night before last night. While I have no hope that anyone will get in touch with the leaflets, if you see something, please call - yes? "Libby nods." Of course, Mr. Knaggs, I'll do that for sure. "Libby had a summer last summer Watch out for the dog of the Knaggs and has since gone to Shorty Gassy or played the dog sitter on weekends. Shorty has since become pretty fond of Libby.

Libby just wants to continue driving, as she stops again: "Mr. Knaggs? It's a nice shock to me that Shorty ran away. I really hope they find him again. "Mr. Knaggs turns around:" Many thanks Libby, but all the doors and windows were locked. I do not think he ran away. "Libby looks dumbfounded," Is that someone's kidnapping Shorty? "Mr. Knaggs nods," It looks like it. "Libby is not sure what to answer:" That's it yes unbelievable! Then I keep my eyes open in any case, "she says and goes on.

On the way to school Libby tells Alex and Popped the whole story. Alex is horrified: "That's a strong piece! A dog hijack here in Sawbuck? That's probably the most exciting thing that ever happened here, is it? "Libby agrees:" I agree. Do you think the old Belbin has anything to do with it? "Alex shakes his head." Oh shit. He is at least 100 years old - how should he have anything to do with it? "Libby continues:" Just think, the old Belbin has the biggest motive. He is constantly complaining about the dog. "

Popped intervenes - somewhat out of breath from cycling - "Libby is right!" Popped gasps: "I trust the old man too." Now he interrupts: "Hey guys, maybe we can stop, if we talk? I get gasp breathing! "The three friends stop and Popped is breathing hard Ok, suppose old Belbin had the faxes thick. What could be more appropriate than to make the dog disappear? "

Alex is not quite sure: "But how should he have done that?" Libby is very excited: "That's exactly what it needs to find out! We'll convict old Belbin! "Popped shakes his head." No, no, no, yesterday I did not make my point clear enough. I do not want to have anything to do with old Belbin! "Libby looks at Popped." Popped, do not you want to pay the old man back? "

Popped thinks for a moment. Then he answers: "Damn, yes, that sounds good. Then I play stick out of the bag! "Libby looks over to Alex:" Are you there too? "Alex hesitates, but then he agrees and extends his hand:" Oh, hell. Then the three musketeers are reunited. "Libby and Popped put their hands on Alex's hand. Then all three cheer at the same time: "One for all and all for one!"

In the afternoon, the three hide in the bushes on the opposite side of the Belbin House. Popped has his binoculars for shading. "I did not know that so many people come by every day!" Says Alex. Libby says, "And we're not the only ones who suspect Belbin," she says. "Did you see how they all shake their heads when they pass Belbin's house?" Suddenly Popped makes a cramped sound: "Ooh, have you seen that? Lisa's mother just passed by and trampled on the flowerbed of old Belbin. "

Alex reaches for the binoculars: "Show me! Fact, not a lie. Everything flat! Libby look. "Alex holds out the binoculars to Libby, but Libby does not take it. What's going on?" Asks Alex. Libby looks thoughtful: "What if we do wrong to old Belbin? If he was not? Everyone seems to think that old Belbin has kidnapped the dog or worse. "

Popped babbles immediately: "Are you kidding me Libby? And if that was the old stick vibrator! Anyone who goes after children, but before all animals has no respect! "Alex holds Popped on the shoulder:" Wait Popped. Libby is right! On television it is always - in doubt for the defendant. "Then he turns to Libby:" Listen to Libby. Even if he was not, we are his best chance of enlightenment. We're only here to find out the truth. "

Popped puffs himself up: "To find out the truth? I think it hacks. I'm here to mop up the old Belbin. "Alex shuts Popper's mouth, still trying to keep talking," Hmmmmmmmmmmmmmm. "Popped frees his mouth," That's good. I understood. We're here to play Samaritan, for an old guy who did not deserve this. Alright Libby. I'm still here! After all, there is a chance that he is guilty and then I want to be there when the handcuffs click. "Alex looks at Libby:" All right Libby? "Libby nods:" All right! Let's find out the truth. "

Slowly dawn breaks and old Belbin was not even visible. "Good that we told our parents that we're having an overnight party with you - Popped," says Alex. "Class idea?" Replies Popped. But Libby is not that enthusiastic: "Well, I did not think it was great to fool my parents." Popped shakes his head: "Nonsense with sauce! We all spend the night together. What was lying there? "Alex looks at Libby:" Well, you have to admit, somehow that makes sense. "Libby nods:" That really makes sense. "Popped interrupts the whole thing:" Pssst, well, rest now! It is dark! The mission begins. "

Exercise

EDUCATION AND WORK

Value: --

Activity: --

Activity: --

Activity: --

Value: --

Activity: --

Activity: --

Activity: --

Chapter 27. A Trip Into Starlight

The night sky holds many wonders and distant mysteries.

For ages, we had gazed up at the stars and looked for answers to our deepest questions, for have used the maps made by the stars to carry us home, and we had told many tales about when mortals became a legend, forever twinkling in the night.

Ask your body to find the most comfortable position.

Lean into that position and scan your whole body for any tension, aches, and pains, anything you might be holding onto physically.

Find those spaces and consciously release them.

Let it all go with your breath.

Relaxation begins with your breath, and throughout this meditation bedtime story, keeping a steady breath will help you find a fully relaxed body, mind, and heart.

You can begin with your breath by simply drawing it into your nostrils and exhaling it out of your nostrils or mouth.

Breathe in slowly, exhale slowly. Inhale...exhale...

Your sense of calm, your serenity, your peace of mind, lives in your breath.

Feel it vacate your body and let all of your muscles turn to jam or jelly.

If your muscles feel hard, soften them.

If your muscles feel tight, loosen them.

Use your breath to find this physical sensation...

Your body is now longer, smoother energy, your muscles are letting go of all of your current stress, and you are now a little more relaxed than you were before.

All of your breathing throughout these moments has taken you farther into your peacefulness and calmness.

All of your inhales and exhales have loosened your grip on the day...

Now that you are a little more relaxed, you can begin to go on your bigger journey into relief and healing.

Your journey begins when you step out of your house.

In your mind, see yourself walking outside of your house and into the night.

The stars are bright.

There are no lights around you.

It is totally black outside except for the starlight.

You feel enveloped by starlight as you look up and see it stretching from one horizon to the other.

The stars are endless, and there isn't a cloud in the sky.

It is clear, and you can see all of the stars in your hemisphere...

Continuing your breath, you welcome the starlight into you as you breathe in, breathing in the feeling of connection to the great unknown, the distant mysteries of the far-off galaxies beyond.

This starlight fills your whole body with each breath and invites you to take a trip to a far-off distant place, somewhere deep within the cosmos...

There is nothing to fear, for you are here to journey.

Your physical body will not be harmed by going so far away.

You can see your journey through the vastness of your inner mind.

When you look down, you know you will not fall.

You are in control of your flight, and you have always flown like this.

It is easy to do and you are relaxed as you take off.

When you look down, you watch the Earth begin to diminish.

The farther you go up to the stars, the smaller the buildings become, the cars, the trains, the highways, the rivers, mountains, and streams...all are becoming smaller and farther away, more distant...

You are falling up...up...up...into the starry night where there is nothing but you and the light of each star twinkling at you.

When you look behind you, Earth is far away, and you are closer to the moon now.

The moon is welcoming and bright.

It feels small compared to the Earth you just came from.

It is big enough for you to sit upon…

You connect to the surface of the moon, and you sit down with your eyes pointing back at the Earth.

You feel as if you can see everything more clearly now.

You are far away from your problems, your cares and worries and you can see your life from the outside looking in—you can feel how different it is to look at yourself and your life from this perspective…

The silvery moonlight feels like it is wrapping itself around you, like an ethereal blanket of security and comfort.

The luminosity is recharging your batteries and helping you to feel rejuvenated and refreshed, like bathing in light…

Your breath comes in, and you can breathe easily here.

You are of the cosmos and so you can survive in this place.

You are ready to carry on and go deeper into the calming serenity of Universal light.

You are going where no one can go on Earth and you are going there with your thoughts, with your subconscious, with your intuition guiding you...

You are going to get ready to leave the moon and travel even farther beyond.

As you stand up on the surface, you feel your body bend at the knees and then push you off the surface.

You begin to float out, away from the moon, being pulled forward into the starry night, beyond Earth, beyond the moon, beyond time...

You can feel yourself getting farther and farther away, and you feel serene, safe and in control.

You are the captain of this interstellar flight.

You are safe and your body is capable of taking this trip.

You are here to find your cosmic truth.

You are here to set yourself free.

You can see your entire reality so clearly from all the way out here, far off into the starry night.

You are here to be, to exist, to enjoy the freedom that exists here.

You are burdened by nothing.

You have no obligations here.

You have only your inner power, your truth, your release from all of your current life problems, and challenges.

You are safe to leave all of your cares and worries in the vastness of the cosmos, in the deep of outer space...

You are free to realize your deepest truth in this place in space.

You are open to all things, and it feels safe and calm.

This is a calm, centered really.

The starlight is holding you closely, protecting you on your journey into the distant realms of space.

You are entering a space that is colorful and big.

A nebula is forming in front of your eyes, like a cosmic waterfall of blue and gold dust speckled with red and green starlight.

This starry cloud of dust opens to you like flower petals blooming on a rose.

You are invited to come closer to it and let yourself fall through it, like a tunnel into another reality.

Getting closer and closer to this massive, smoky, rainbow, you begin to feel pulled into it softly.

It is gentle and calm, and you are not in a hurry, out here in the great beyond...

The nebula surrounds you softly, gently.

It begins to turn into a tunnel that your body can float through.

You are not sure where the tunnel will lead, but you are calm and relaxed.

You don't need to know.

You are full of the power of the cosmos, and you are at peace in your mind and your body.

You allow your body to just glide through the nebula tunnel, feeling open to whatever lies beyond...

You are transported through the tunnel until you feel your body sitting on a sandy shore...you take a look around at this space, a wide, vast landscape on another planet, somewhere in a distant galaxy.

You can feel the softness of the sand.

It is different from Earth's sand, softer, finer, blue-green in places, and splotches of yellow and red in others...

The air is fresh here.

You can breathe easily.

You feel relaxed and calm, curiously taking in the place you have found through the tunnel.

You can feel the air is warm but not too hot.

You can feel a soft breeze that brings you into contact with a beautiful scent on the air.

There are strange and exotic flowers and plants that look foreign, alien to you.

You are drawn to their unique qualities and colors, like nothing you have ever seen on Earth before...

Sitting here in this place, you are able to feel the calmness of your mind, body, and heart.

You are in total peace and centeredness.

You stand up and take a deep breathe in, pulling in all of the wonderful serenity of this far-off distant shore.

The nebula gas returns and pulls you in, as if it never left you, as if it was always there, waiting for you to return home...

You are ready to transcend space and time once more and travel back through the tunnel.

You find your way through the nebula tunnel with ease and grace, moving slowly, gently.

You are drawing closer and closer to the space where you entered the tunnel, and as you come out of it, you find yourself back in the vastness of outer space, covered in starlight.

You are pulled from the nebula, floating back through the cosmos the way that you came, retracing your steps through the ethereal realms of the stars.

Each breath you take in and exhale will push you forward to your destination.

Each inhale gives you the life force you need to propel yourself back home.

Each exhale gets you closer to your healing and relief, letting it all go and leaving it way out here in space...

You are much closer to home now because you can see the moon again.

You are narrowing in on the moon, and you decide to take a break here before making the final trip home to your house.

You float toward the surface of the moon and gracefully land, finding a comfortable spot to sit and absorb the luminosity of the moon's surface.

You can feel the earnest efforts of all people to lead a good life and search for a deeper truth.

Looking out upon the Earth from this place, you remind yourself that even the biggest problems you face are little compared to the energy of all life in the Universe.

Here you can feel refreshed, relaxed, the calm of mind and body.

You stand up on the moon's surface and prepare to launch.

You push yourself off of the surface and glide slowly and peacefully toward the Earth.

You are following the same path you took to get up to the stars.

It will take you right back to your house where you stood outside and looked up at the starlight...

You are getting closer and closer to the Earth's surface, and the moon is a distant friend again.

You can feel yourself being pulled in the right direction.

You are not in a hurry.

You are not picking up speed.

You are gently floating, flying home slowly, delicately, peacefully.

The mountains and trees, the rivers and streams are beginning to become larger, closer, as you slowly descend back to the surface of your home planet.

Exercise

PHYSICAL HEALTH

Value: --

Activity: --

Activity: --

Activity: --

Value: --

Activity: --

Activity: --

Activity: --

Chapter 28. The Award-Winning Story

Everyone at Jefferson High School knew who Billy was. He had made a point to start his career as a journalist since he was just a little kid. In fifth grade, Billy passed around fliers telling the students what books were banned in their school library.

A few years after that, he was in the club closest to publishing: the yearbook committee. If it hadn't been for the teacher supervisor and the other students, that yearbook would have been filled with personal details about the students throughout their pictures. He thought the yearbook shouldn't just be about the pictures, but who these students were.

Billy had honed a skill for talking with people and getting information from them; he collected many interesting tidbits about the students: which ones didn't like the controversial math teacher, which ones were moving away, which ones had secrets they would rather not share.

Back in those days, people thought he was just having an intimate chat with them, not trying to put their deepest secrets into print. Now that Billy and all his classmates were in high school, they knew better than to share anything personal with him.

Jefferson High School was the largest high school in the state, giving Billy quite a different experience from the tiny junior high he had attended. On the one hand, it meant there was no shortage of juicy info to get inside that building, but on the other hand, the sheer size made that info all the more difficult to sift through.

Now Billy was in tenth grade, and he was still on his never-ending quest to prove his value as a journalist. He could feel the suspicious stares from people, but they didn't bother him.

Billy had ambitions and dreams, and he was willing to do whatever it took to achieve them. The way he saw it, the reputation he had in high school, was insignificant compared to what he would do with his career for the rest of his life.

It wasn't only his reputation that made people wary of Billy. His appearance gave off some signs he was not someone to be trusted. As if he were some kind of detective, he wore a tweed jacket that looked baggy on his tall, slim build. He tended to wear dark jeans as if he were trying to hide in the shadows. Most suspicious of all was his thick pair of eyeglasses that made it impossible to look at his eyes to see what he was thinking.

The reputation had followed him from his younger year until today, and he knew it wasn't going to leave him behind until he graduated. But while Billy was the kind of kid who people talked about, he didn't pay mind to any of it. He was always too busy with whatever investigation he was currently undergoing.

That day, he had gotten detention on purpose so he could ask the detention to monitor some questions. He had heard a rumor that some of the kids who came here every day were actually doing it to get out of athletic commitments.

It was a titillating piece of gossip, to say the least. Athletes were worshipped at Jefferson, and if there were kids who were avoiding practices and games, that was something worth looking into.

Billy flipped through the pages of his book casually, eyeing the detention monitor, Ms. Helgen, over the cover. He didn't want it to seem like he was up to anything. Even though people always assumed he was, Billy still always found a way to make people think they weren't one of the people he was using.

Getting her attention was no easy feat. She was preoccupied with the box of crackers she was eating in front of everyone. No one else was allowed to eat during detention, so it was a slightly cruel thing to do. Billy tried to catch her gaze with an innocent-sounding question.

"Ms. Helgen, what time is it?" he asked her. He thought it should sound like an innocuous question, because everyone had to put their phones on the table at the beginning of detention, and no one wore watches.

Ms. H knew what the kids thought about Billy, but she was so engrossed in her snack, she didn't even notice his question until he repeated himself twice.

That was when Ms. Helgen realized the detention was supposed to end ten minutes ago. She dismissed the whole class, leaving no one in the room, but Billy.

Since she ran out of chicken crackers, she had no good excuse for not listening to Billy when he tried to speak with her after detention.

"Trying to cause problems as usual?" she asked him. "I hate to be the one to break it to you, but real life isn't like a movie. You're not going to find anything worth writing about in this school. This place is as boring as it gets."

"A place where no one thinks there is scandal is the perfect place for a scandal to hide," Billy argued. He pulled out his notebook to write down any potential information that Ms. H could give him. "I've heard people saying that some of the athletes in detention today had practices to go to. Why would they stay back from practice?"

The real question he wanted to ask was what they got into trouble for. Since he thought the behavior itself was suspicious on its face, he didn't think it likely that it was just a coincidence. They had to be getting in trouble to get out of these commitments on purpose — what he really wanted to know was why.

Oddly, asking the question directly wasn't how he expected to get an answer. He saw this as a way to make it clear what his intentions were in his investigation. Ms. H probably had very little information on her own, but she might have some smaller tidbits that could lead him in the right direction.

Billy had picked up this strategy from his growing body of experience of interviewing people. When he made it clear what he was searching for, it made them less defensive.

They didn't feel like he was hiding something when he came right out with things. But when they let their guards down like this that gave him the opportunity to ask smaller questions that might get him to the answers he was really searching for.

"This is just what the other teachers have warned me about you. You're nothing but trouble," Ms. H said. "I don't want to get involved in whatever this is. I just want to go home and watch my documentaries."

This was no issue. Billy never expected to get anything from that question, after all. It would have been worse if he hadn't made his intentions clear, and she was on edge the whole time. Now, he could ask her something she might actually be able to answer.

"What are they in here for?" he asked.

"The same minor offenses as you. Kids these days can't even get to school on time. When they show up late three days in the same term, they get detention. Just like you did. Although, it is rare to see any of you in here, including you." Ms. H looked at him. "You didn't really come in here just to talk to me, did you? If that's the case, you're not going to get anything better than what you've already got. So you might as well keep your expectations low. But Harold and Terrence are in detention today and Saturday. That's as deep as this gets."

"Of course not. I've been having trouble waking up on time in the mornings, that's all," he said, but Ms. H didn't look so sure. It didn't matter. He had already gotten everything he was going to get out of this teacher, and it wasn't much.

All he did learn was that these athletes were going to detention for coming to school late. Not only that, but like him, these were not students who normally went to detention. It may have been coincidental, but too many things lined up for it to be likely that they didn't get detention on purpose. There had to be some scandal at the Athletic Department.

This was terrific news for him because all he wanted to do was publish a good story in the school paper, the Presidential Chronicle. He didn't care what it took. The only stories he got to write were stale, boring ones that no one read. Nobody wanted to read a story about how flooding affected the parking lot. Nobody wanted to read a story about how parts of the core curriculum had changed.

The truth was, Billy wasn't happy with just getting this one story. He wanted prolonged fame from everyone who went to this school; Billy wanted to be a part of the conversation in the community.

He simply wasn't happy blending into the background. He wanted to be known as a capable and driven individual, and he also wanted to have some accomplishments to speak of when he applied to prestigious schools in his junior year. Billy knew that he needed to plan ahead.

His investigation of detention hadn't been especially fruitful, so he decided to go right to the Athletic office and see what he could dig up. Billy would still have to be quick about it because he didn't have his driver's license yet, so his mother was coming to pick him up soon after detention.

The last time he went to the Athletic Office, he had tried to find out if the wrestling team had been using PEDs to succeed in competitions, which turned out to be a false lead.

He could only hope there was someone different at the office today who wouldn't remember him from last year. Even if that turns out to be the case, though, he would be able to pull this off.

He packed up his things in his back-up and started the long walk to the Athletics Office on the other side of the building. There were few people roaming the hallways at this time of day; everyone had either gone home, they were with their teams outside, or they were in the auditorium with the performing arts clubs.

Exercise

RECREATION/LEISURE

Value: --

Activity: --------------------------------------

Activity: --------------------------------------

Activity: --------------------------------------

Value: --

Activity: --------------------------------------

Activity: --------------------------------------

Activity: --------------------------------------

Chapter 29. Quiet Night In The Forest

The moment you feel ready to take a journey into the forest at night, you will lay your body down and find comfort in the room where you are the calmest, most peaceful, and relaxed.

You will want to make sure that you are warm, covered with blankets, or wearing warm clothing.

Make your body feel as relaxed as possible so that you can go deeper into your thoughts and mind.

Finding your relaxed position, begin to breathe deeply.

Notice your chest lifting, your abdomen extending.

Act upon the breath as slowly and steadily as you are able and hold for a count of one...two...three...release the breath as slowly and as steadily as you brought into your chest and body.

Again, with the feeling of total peace, pull oxygen into your chest and abdomen, filling the space within you as slowly and as steadily as you can...and hold the breath for a count of one...two...three...and release it as slowly as you pulled it into your body.

Your breathing can continue this way, or as it feels the most relaxing and calming to you.

Let your breath simply exist and do what it must to help you foster your serenity and sense of calm.

Your breath is pushing away any tension you may be feeling right now.

Your breath is helping you connect more fully to your body and your mind.

Your breath is sending you on a path of rest and rejuvenation.

Let your breath carry you there, quietly, slowly, steadily...

As you begin to sink into your mattress or cushions, wherever your body is lying down, you are going to begin to take a journey into the quiet of a forest at night, but first, you must get there.

The forest is not far.

It is a deeper part of you, a place inside of you that you can journey to when your body is at peace, and your breathing is relaxed.

Your inner world is made by you, and this quiet forest is a haven for you to become full of peaceful thoughts and empowered dreams to help you heal from the inside out.

Whatever you may be suffering from at this time in your life, sleeplessness, anxiety, worry…depression, frustration, self-doubt…whatever you are struggling with is going to be cleared in the quiet forest in the night.

All you have to do is find your way there from the comfort of this position you are laying in now.

You will get there easily-as your body becomes more relaxed through your breathing, as you allow yourself to let go of anything you might be clutching onto from the outside world, from your experiences, from your past…

Every breath will take you deeper into your relaxed body and state of mind.

You are here to travel into your subconscious mind and find a quiet space to release any fears, any doubts, your cares, and worries.

The quiet night in the forest is where you will go to heal these parts of you, these thoughts and feelings, these attitudes and beliefs...

The quiet of the forest realm will give you the permission and security you need to rest and dream without worry or grief.

All you have to do is relax more deeply into this position you are lying, your breath, relaxing into your deeper sense of self, falling deeper and deeper into the quiet night that surrounds you...

As you enter this space, you begin by noticing that your feet bare.

You look down and notice your bare feet standing on the ground.

The ground is safe and secure.

You feel comfortable here, with your feet bare, and you know that when you take a step forward, you will be walking towards your relief.

Your feet begin to carry you in that direction.

It is dark all around you, but for the silver moonlight that you can feel blanketing this landscape.

As you begin to notice what surrounds you in this space, you can feel the forest calling to you.

It is not far away, and you can see the shadow and silhouette of the trees and the ridge that the forest covers on the horizon...

Their silent, quiet lights are friendly and guiding you forward on your path to the center of the quiet night in the forest.

They are everywhere, flashing warm, yellow-orange lights from their bodies, slowly dancing about the fresh, pine-scented forest...

You hear the soft tinkling again, and you begin to calmly follow it through the thickness of trees as the fireflies continue their merry dance of quiet light.

You follow the tinkling sound, like little bells or chimes being tickled by the night air of the wood.

There is a warmth to this sound, and you know that it is special and good, that it is guiding to just the right place...

You feel the soft, mossy earth beneath your feet, like a growing, velvet carpet that stretches out in every direction, comforting every footstep you take as you follow the tinkling bells further into the forest.

The only sound is the sound of your bare feet against the soft moss and the tinkling bell.

Everything else is soft, serene, gentle, and bathes in moonlight...

The forest is happy you are here, happy you have come.

It wants you to find peacefulness and relief.

The forest exists deep within you to offer you comfort from stress and worry relief from grief, and suffering.

The forest is here to hold your hand as you walk toward your destination of deep relaxation and a peaceful night's sleep...

Everywhere you look, you see glorious trees, fireflies, and the soft, pale moonlight touching everything it can.

You look ahead of you as the tinkling seems a little closer to you.

You feel a warmth and a glow from somewhere far away. The distant glow asks you to come closer.

You know that it is safe and that there is friendliness in all parts of this quiet forest at night.

You can hear the tinkling bells more now.

The sound is coming from the warm glow at the center of a copse of trees, not too distant from where you are right now.

The fireflies are swimming through the air toward this place of light, and the bells are harmonious as they chime...

You find yourself close to the outside of the circle of trees and hiding behind one.

You look into the center of the warm and soothing glow.

At the center of the copse of trees is a beam of light, pouring out from the soil in a shaft or beam pointed up towards the starlight.

You cannot tell if the beam of light is coming from the cosmos and the stars, or from the warm center of the Earth...

Above the beam of light, high up in the trees, you notice a treehouse.

You see a set of steps to climb up to the treehouse at the top of the tree it is sitting in, and you notice a small set of wind chimes dangling from the treehouse roof.

There is the sound that I called you to this center.

There is the sacred space that has been calling out you since you entered the forest...

Coming out from behind the tree, you enter the cops and walk toward the shaft of light glowing from the center and beaming up to the heavens through past the treehouse.

You are here to resolve all of your tension and stress, all of your anxiety and worry and doubt.

This circle of trees, this shaft of light, this is where you cleanse yourself of all of the thoughts and emotions that keep you feeling far away from rest, that keeps you locked in cycles of doubt and worry.

You will now step forward into the beam of light and allow yourself to be bathed in it.

This light is coming from high above from the cosmic life flow of the distant planets and stars.

This light is coming from deep within the Earth.

It is all connected, going up and down all at once.

And now, as you are stepping into this light, you are able to feel the total purity of mind and spirit that comes from true relief...

You have all that you need right here, right now, in this beam of light.

You have everything you will need to find peace of mind and body and get the rest that you deserve.

You no longer have to carry any burdens or fears.

You can release them into this beam of light and let them return to the cosmic flow of all things.

It will take care of that energy for you.

You can give it what ails you, depresses you, keeps you feeling afraid at night, all of that can go directly into this beam of light.

As you stand here, feel this warm glowing beam flow through the soles of your bare feet, up through your ankles and your legs.

See and feel this light go through your knees and thighs, up through your hips and pelvis...

Follow this light up through your torso, filling your abdomen, your organs, and your bloodstream.

See the shaft of light going into your arms and hands, your chest, neck, shoulders.

See the light filling your headspace.

This light is a part of you, and you are a part of it—it is the cosmic life force of both Earth and Stars, and it is here to relieve you of your doubts and fears.

You are alone in this light in this circle of trees and all you have to do is breathe and watch it fill your whole being with soft comfort and powerful awakening...

You are letting go now of all of the worries and cares of your mind.

You can see the light reflecting off of the trees that are encircling you.

They are wise, old, and powerful.

They are full of healing light and energy and will continue to hold you and keep you safe in the quiet night in the forest.

When you are ready, you notice the steps that will lead you to the treetop and into the treehouse.

Full of light, you decide to climb up to the top and into the warm and welcoming home high up in the trees…

A good night's rest.

Exercise

DAILY ACTIVITIES

Today's Date: _____

TIME ACTIVITY   ENJOYMENT (0–10)
        IMPORTANCE (0–10)

Chapter 30. Count Neighbors

Piotr Mijáilich Vashon was in a very bad mood: his sister, a single girl, had run away with Valsecchi, who was a married man. Trying to drive away the deep depression that had taken hold of him and that left him neither at home nor in the countryside, he called to his aid the feeling of justice, his honest convictions (because he had always been a supporter of freedom in the countryside!), but this did not help, and each time, against his will, he came to the same conclusion: that the stupid babysitter, that is, that his sister had done wrong and that Valsecchi had abducted her. And this was horrible.

The mother did not leave her room, the babysitter spoke in a low voice and did not stop sighing, the aunt expressed constant desire to leave, and her bags were already taken out to the anteroom, and they were taken back to her room. Inside the house, in the courtyard, and in the garden, there was a silence such that there seemed to be a deceased. The aunt, the servitude, and even the music's, as it seemed to Piotr Mijáilich, looked at him with an enigmatic and perplexed expression, as if they wanted to say: «They have seduced your sister, why do you stay with your arms crossed? » He also reproached himself for his inactivity, although he did not know what it was, in fact, what he should do.

Thus, six days passed. The seventh - a Sunday, after lunch - a man on horseback brought a letter. The address - «To your Excel. Anna Nikolayev Iváshina »- was written with familiar female characters. Piotr Mijáilich thought he saw in the envelope, in the characters and in the half-written word, "Excel.", something provocative, liberal. And women's liberalism is stubborn, ruthless, cruel...

"He will prefer death before making a concession to his miserable mother, before asking for forgiveness," thought Piotr Mijáilich when he went in search of his mother with the letter in hand.

She was in bed but dressed. When he saw the son, he sat up impulsively and, fixing the gray hair that had come out of the cap, asked with a quick phrase: -

What is there? What's up?

"He sent ..." said the son, handing him the letter.

Zina's name and even the pronoun "she" were not pronounced in the house. Zina was spoken impersonally: "has sent," "is gone," ... The mother recognized the daughter's writing, and her face, disengaged, became unpleasant. Gray hair escaped from the cap again.

-Do not! He said, pushing his hands away as if the letter had burned his fingers. No, no, never! For nothing in the world!

The mother broke into hysterical sobs caused by pain and embarrassment; He seemed to want to read the letter, but pride prevented him. Piotr Mijáilich realized that he must open it and read it aloud, but suddenly he felt dominated by anger as he had never known. He ran to the patio and shouted at the man who had brought the letter: -

Say there will be no answer! There will be no answer! Say it like that, animal!

And then he shattered the letter. Then tears came to his eyes and, feeling cruel, guilty, and unhappy, and he went to the countryside.

He was only twenty-seven years old, but he was already fat, dressed as old men, in very loose suits, and suffered from dyspnea. He already had all the inclinations of the single landowner. He did not fall in love, and he did not think about getting married and only loved his mother, his sister, the babysitter, and the gardener Vasilis. He liked to eat well, take a nap, and talk about politics and high subjects... He had finished studies at the University at the time, but now he looked at this as if it had been an inevitable burden for young people from eighteen to twenty-five. At least, the ideas that now roamed every day through his head had nothing in common with the University or with what he had studied in it.

It was hot in the countryside, and everything was calm, like announcing rain. The forest exhaled slight steam and a pungent smell of pine and decayed leaves. Piotr Mijáilich often stopped to wipe the sweat from his forehead. He checked his wheat fields of autumn and spring, toured the alfalfa field, and a couple of times, in a forest clearing, frightened a partridge with his pellets. And to all this, I kept thinking that such an unbearable situation could not last forever and that they should put an end to it in one way or another. Anyway, in a stupid, absurd way, but it had to end.

"But how? What to do? He wondered, looking at the sky and the trees as if imploring his help.

But the sky and the trees were silent. Honest convictions were useless, and common sense told him that the lacerating problem could only have a stupid solution and that the scene with the man who had brought the letter would not be the last of this genre. He was afraid to think about what could still happen.

He turned home when the sun was setting. Now it seemed to him that the problem could not have any solution. It was impossible to accept the accomplished fact, but neither could it not be accepted, and there was no average solution. When, with his hat in his hand and making air with his handkerchief, he was marching along the road, and there were a couple of vests left at home, he heard a bell ringing behind him. It was a very nice set of bells and bells that produced a jingle like crystals. It could only be Demoski, the chief of the district police, a former Hussar officer who had wasted his property and his health, a sick man, a distant relative of Piotr Mijáilich. He had great confidence with the Vashon and felt great admiration and paternal love for Zina.

"I'm going home," he said when he reached the height of Piotr Mijáilich. Climb, I'll take it.

He was smiling jovially; it was clear that he did not know about Zina. Perhaps they had told him, and he had not believed it. Piotr Mijáilich felt in a violent situation.

"I celebrate it," he stammered, flushing, to the point that tears came, and not knowing what a lie to say. I'm very happy, "he continued, trying to smile, "but... Zina is gone, and mom is sick.

-What a pity! Said the police chief, looking thoughtfully at Piotr Mijáilich. And I who planned to spend the evening with you... Where have Zinnia Mijáilovna gone?

-To the house of the Sinofsky, from there, it seems that he wanted to go to the monastery. I do not know for sure.

The police chief said something else and turned around. Piotr Mijáilich went home thinking horrified at what the police chief would feel when he knew the truth. He imagined it, and under this impression, he entered the house.

"Help me, Lord, help me ..." he thought.

In the dining room, having tea, there was the only aunt. "Your mother hasn't eaten today," said Aunt. "You, Petr Usha, you should pay attention." Letting ourselves starve will not relieve our misfortune.

It seemed absurd to Piotr Mijáilich that the aunt mingles in matters that were none of her business and made her departure depend on the fact that Zina had left. He wanted to tell her an insolence, but he held back. And when he contained himself, he warned that the opportune time had come to act, that he was unable to suffer any longer. Or do something right now, or fall to the ground screaming and nodding. He imagined that Valsecchi and Zina, both liberal and self-satisfied, kissed under a maple, and all the weight and grudge that had accumulated in him during the seven days turned over Valsecchi.

He jumped to his feet and quickly stepped out of the dining room. In the stable, the administrator's horse was saddled. He rode on it and galloped in search of Valsecchi.

A true storm had unleashed in his soul. I felt the need to do something that came out of the ordinary, tremendous, even if I had to regret it during my entire life. Call miserable Valsecchi, slap him, and then challenge him? But Valsecchi was not one of those who grieve, and, feeling crossed out as miserable and receiving the slap, all he would be to feel more miserable and more secluded in himself. These unfortunate and submissive people are the most unbearable beings, the most difficult to deal with. Everything about them goes unpunished. When the unfortunate man, in response to a deserved reproach, looks with eyes that reflect the awareness of his guilt, smiles painfully, and meekly approaches his head, it seems that justice itself is unable to raise its hand against it.

"Is the same. I will shake a whip before her and tell her a few rudeness's, "Piotr Mijáilich decided.

He rode through his forest and his wastelands and imagined the way Zina, justifying his action, would speak of women's rights, personal freedom and that it was absolutely the same to marry for the Church or for the civil. He would discuss, as a woman he was, things he did not understand. And I would probably ask him: «What do you have to do with all this? What right do you have to intrude?

—Yes, I don't have any rights —grain Piotr Mijáilich— But the better... The more rude it is, the less right it has, the better.

It was stifling heat. Clouds of mosquitoes flew very low, flush with the ground, and in the barren, the faults cried mournfully. Piotr Mijáilich crossed its borders and continued galloping across a completely smooth field. He had traveled this road many times and knew every thicket, until the last-ditch. What is the distance between two lights, looked like a dark rock, was a red church; you could imagine it to the last detail, even the plastering of the portal and the calves that always grazed in its enclosure. On the right, a versa of the church blacked the grove of Count Koltóvich. And after the grove, the lands of Valsecchi began.

Behind the church and the count's grove was a huge cloud, which occasionally was illuminated by pale lightning.

"There is! Thought Piotr Mijáilich. Help me, sir!"

The horse soon showed signs of fatigue, and Piotr Mijáilich himself felt fatigued. The cloud looked at him angrily, as if advising him to return home. He felt a certain fear.

«I will show you that you are not right! -He tried to instill courage- They will say that this is free love, personal freedom, but freedom is in abstention, and not in subordination to passions. His is depravity and not freedom! » tail.

Exercise

Evidence for my thought Evidence against my thought

---------------------------   ---------------------------

---------------------------   ---------------------------

---------------------------   ---------------------------

---------------------------   ---------------------------

Chapter 31. Animal Dreams

In every good fable, you will find an animal that helps to tell a story.

In every place in nature, you find the whimsical and ethereal beasts who call Mother Earth home, just like you.

For centuries, many different peoples have looked to animals for messages of truth, divination, omens of things to come, and ways to feel protected, brave and safe.

Your personal spirit animal may not be the same every time you meditate on them.

Sometimes, an animal spirit guide will come to you to help foster growth and change in new ways.

All animals are symbolic of something, and all of your experiences with this mediation will give you the messages that you are needing right now on your path.

Look to the animal spirits for their symbolic messages and what they might represent to you as you go on your meditation journey.

Ask your animal spirit guide to come to you through your dreams to show you a path that is just right for you…right now.

You may have the same spirit animal come to you many times, or you may meet a variety of animal spirit guides on your path.

For whatever reason, the animal that comes to you today is the one with the answers for your journey.

You can find friendship and take comfort in your animal guides and learn from them what magic awaits you when you enter into an animal dream.

For this guided meditation, find a comfortable and relaxing position to enjoy as you relax your body and mind.

You can lie on the floor, in your bed, on some cushions…anywhere that feels safe, relaxing, and calming.

You may want to fall asleep, and that's okay.

You are going to find your relief through a walk through the kingdom of animals.

To begin, find your inhale.

Relax into yourself as you breathe in deeply and let go of your day or your week as you let your breath out.

Inhale slowly, relaxing into your body a little further...and exhale away the last few hours, days, weeks...anything that is in need of release...

Inhale gently, slowly...give your body all of the fresh air it needs to feel refreshed and relieved...exhale slowly, steadily, letting out the tension and stress of life, giving yourself permission to simply let go and relax.

Continue your breathing in this way for several breath cycles...

You are more relaxed now.

You have a heaviness to your muscles because you know you don't need to go anywhere or do anything.

Let go of any worries and cares that you should be accomplishing something else right now.

Your only purpose at this time is to rest and relax.

You can wander freely in the animal kingdom from this place of true relaxation.

Your body and your mind are free to go on a journey to a long-forgotten land where the elders whispered stories of the great beasts and birds of legend, the ones who told the tales of strength and courage, of tenderness and patience, of dedication or perseverance...

The animals of the ancient world are similar to the ones you see walking around today.

In the landscape of your mind, on your journey into deeper awareness, your animal spirit guide can resemble anything at all...any color...any size...any shape...any texture.

Your dream animal is your companion into the dream world, who will lead you toward a sense of trust with yourself and the power you hold within.

As you inhale again, breathe into a distant place...a landscape far off in your dreamland.

Look around this place and notice what it looks like.

What are the features you notice? Is it a desert, a lake, a forest?

Are you on an island covered in jungle, or in a tropical rainforest?

Are you somewhere near the ocean?

Explore your landscape in your mind for a moment and let yourself wander through this hidden realm of your subconscious mind...

How hot or cold is it?

Is it cloudy and raining, or warm and sunny?

Do you feel a breeze or a strong wind?

Focus on the details of your landscape.

Allow it to truly come to life for you in your mind...

As you feel yourself becoming more relaxed and in tune with your inner world, you notice a path.

The path is made for you to follow it.

The path is leading you closer to your destination and your animal guide.

For some, your animal guide may have already shown up for you, and that's okay.

The animal guide will still ask you to walk this path, and it will walk with you...

If you have not seen the animal come forward for you yet, do not struggle to make it appear.

It will come to you when you are in the right moment of relaxation and relief.

You will now begin to walk on this path, one step at a time.

Use your imagination to give life to the world you have created in your mind.

You are an explorer, and you have the power to imagine the detail of this place as you walk through it.

The path is not straight.

It winds and bends and takes you over and under, out and through, around and behind.

It circles through this landscape in ways only you can see.

Your journey will begin again once you have encountered this creature.

You feel yourself getting nearer as the fog begins to lift, and you can see more clearly.

As the smoke clears, relax, and just look.

Don't tell yourself what it is going to be; just see it.

There on the path in front of you, right now, is your animal spirit guide who will escort you on your journey.

The fog is fully lifted and the animal is here before you, awaiting you on the road.

Take a few moments to observe your animal friend.

Let them take shape. See the details of their shape, form, texture, and size.

Notice what kind of fur or feather or scales they might have.

Notice the shape of their eyes, their nose, and their mouth.

Do they have whiskers?

A beak?

A snout?

Show yourself fully what your animal spirit guide looks like and let the vision of their shape sit with you for a moment before you move forward...

The animal that has come to you, no matter whether it is snake or bear, octopus or hummingbird, squirrel or pigeon, it will have an important message for you as you drift further off into sleep and find your deepest comfort.

Feel it, sense its energy with your inner mind.

Show yourself how it feels to be closer to this creature in your imagination...

As you bond with your animal companion, give them an opportunity to show you a message.

Anything that they do could be helpful for you, and it is up to you to interpret what that message is.

Don't overthink it.

Just let it come to you naturally.

It might not come until tomorrow or a few days from now, and that's okay.

You may need time to reflect on the mystical purpose of your animal guide...

Continue to inhale deeply, relaxing into this moment, into feeling out the power of your animal guide.

Allow that essence or spirit to circulate within and around you.

Let this being, give you the opportunity to see something more clearly, to direct your focus in a new way, to take comfort in a hidden answer to a long-asked question...

You will begin to feel the opening of your gift from this animal guide as you continue forward into your dreams tonight.

For now, you can continue to travel through your mindscape with your new friend.

Let the animal pick which way you are going to go, and follow.

See what direction the creature will take and trust that they have your best interests at heart.

They are here to help you find what you are looking for...

Your guide knows where to take you and you can trust them to keep you safe and secure.

Your guide is leading you into new territory, a place you have never been or seen in your mind before.

You are close together; they never stray too far from your side.

This creature has gotten you closer to something you value, something of great importance to you in your life.

You can feel that there is something opening inside of you, something that you have needed to be shown by a trusted friend and guide...

Your animal guide is letting you know with their own energy and actions that you need to stop on the path and wait.

They want you to listen to your heart for a few moments so that you are ready to see what they have wanted to show you.

As you inhale and exhale for a few breath cycles, connect to your heart center.

Breathe into your soul, your mind, your body.

Let the breath fill you with warmth and compassion for your own unique life story...

The animal wants you to see what comes next on your path.

Your guide wants to show you what you need to be thinking about, focusing on, realizing.

They are asking you to stand tall and connect to yourself fully so that you can look even deeper into your heart for answers...for the truth...

They are ready to help you forward now.

You are back on the footpath, and the fog has returned.

You can hardly see through it, but your animal guide is with you now leading you forward.

You have nothing to fear...

Your guide disappears into the fog as you continue to slowly walk the path.

You feel and see the fog lifting now, and your animal friend is waiting for you here, guarding a sacred doorway that leads to your heart center.

You step forward to the door in the middle of the path that seems to lead into nothing and nowhere.

You lay your hand on the knob and turn it.

Your animal guide is by your side and can help you find your way through.

The door is open now.

See what lies on the other side.

You may not be ready to step through the doorway yet, but you are certainly welcome to just look within and discover your truth.

Stand tall with your animal guide beside you and let yourself look deep within your heart...your mind...your soul.

This is what your friend wanted to show you.

This is what you are being guided to see.

Take it in as you take in another few breaths in and out.

Spend time noticing what this means to you.

When you are ready, you can step through the doorway with your animal companion by your side. Let them guide you further now into the world of dreams.

Exercise

What is a more accurate and helpful way of looking at the situation?

Chapter 32. Taking Flight In Dreamland

Almost all of us have had a dream that we are flying.

Sometimes you have wings.

Sometimes you are just gliding through the air like a superhero.

Often times, when we take flight in our dreams, it is symbolic of freedom and a way for us to become connected to letting go of our fears about life in general.

Flying has been described in the legends of old myths and folktales describing a flying person as having special powers.

These tales will always lead you to a form of self-discovery in which you take control of your journey, your destiny.

You are the captain and you know exactly where to fly, how high, and when to land.

Planting your feet on the solid ground all day can be hard, especially if you have a challenging or difficult situation or people in your life, or if you have a hard time processing your feelings and emotions.

Guided meditations and creative visualization are a huge part of how many enlightened people find their way to wholeness.

Your inner journey is just as valuable, meaningful, and important as your inner one.

When you follow your journey forward and trust yourself to fly in the right direction for yourself, then the stresses of life naturally fall away, and you can find peace, harmony, and balance with your whole life. So take a moment to connect with this positive notion.

Find your comfort zone, and let yourself fall into freely.

You are here to enjoy your life journey, not stress out about it all of the time.

You are here to have a purpose that is meaningful to you, not worry about whether or not you are doing a good enough job, or if you are successful enough.

You have always been and always are enough, and when you acknowledge that truth... that's when you can really fly.

Find your most comfortable position.

Find the parts of your body that feel restless or tense and shake them out.

Shake out any part of your body that has felt motionless for far too long.

Shake off anything that you might have absorbed from another person today, or from a challenging experience.

Shake off all of the drama that finds you when you are trying to find your peace of mind...

Inhale deeply and enjoy the way it feels to have control over your breath.

Exhale slowly and appreciate the way it feels to let go of something physically from your body.

Inhale slowly again, rejoicing in the fresh air that fills you up.

Exhale slowly and feel gratitude that you have come to this place of self-healing, to totally bond with your own creative inspiration and thoughts, to become even more closely connected to your inner self, free of drama, free of critique...no judgments.

Your breath has helped your body feel more relaxed.

You are sinking more deeply into your comfort and relaxation.

You are finding it easier to breathe naturally and smoothly.

You are feeling content just to be present here, taking good care of yourself, giving yourself all of the love, attention, and devotion that you need right now...

There are no rules on your inner journey.

All you have to do is appreciate your creative ability to see more clearly from your inner world.

How would you like to feel right now?

Do you feel the way you look in your reflection within your mind?

Do you look the way that you hope to feel?

As you gaze at your inner reflection, show yourself how you want to appear to yourself.

Give yourself the costume or uniform, the style or outfit that best suits how you want to feel within tonight.

You can change your hairstyle.

You can wear something you would normally never choose to put on in public.

Take a few moments as you breathe to appreciate the world you know in your mind.

You can be all of yourself here.

Allow yourself to appear the way you would like to feel right now...

You are going to feel like this for the rest of your guided meditation.

This is your world, and you can look and dress; however, you see fit.

You can change your outfit anytime you want to.

You can become whatever you really are deep down inside.

You might become an animal or a tree.

You might become a warrior or a princess.

You might become something that this world has never know before.

Enjoy the work of dressing yourself to fly.

When you are ready, inhale deeply...hold the breath for a count of three...and steadily release the breath from your body...

You are climbing up a staircase now.

It is made of stone, and it is carved as a spiral, going higher and higher.

It looks like the stairs within an ancient castle.

The castle is a part of your subconscious mind.

It is a place you can come to any time you need to dress yourself the way you want to or hope to feel inside and out...

The stairs are taking you up to the top of the castle.

When you get to the rooftop, you are able to walk out onto it.

The castle overlooks a great and vast kingdom.

It is familiar to you.

You have traveled here before.

As you look out over the land, you can point out to yourself other places you have already been: in a meadow, in a forest, by the ocean on a ship, in the clouds, by a river, in a garden of wonders...

This place holds the secret truth of you and your inner journey.

The landscape is wholly yours, and you can be anything here and do anything you want to help yourself find your truth and purpose.

It is where you will return as you quest for deeper meaning in your life, as you seek to know who you really are, deep down inside...

Standing on the castle roof, taking in the inner world of your mind, you are now able to take a new journey.

Your inner wisdom is what can help you find what you need to see right now, to help you relax and find peace of mind and inner calm.

You can let yourself find the right path when you trust yourself that you already know the answers.

You already know how to solve all of your problems and you can find it all right here in this inner kingdom of your body, mind, heart, and soul...

To take flight, all you have to do is face the world you have created in your thoughts and mind.

Take a moment to breathe and relax into this visual journey.

Take a moment to connect with your breath again and let yourself feel that moment before you take flight...

Stepping closer to the roof's edge, imagine you are outstretching your arms like they are wings, stretching far out to either side of you.

Underneath you are just castle grounds...or is it a waterfall that leads through a great misty fog that goes to another place in your kingdom?

When you look down, you see not the grounds of a castle, but a portal into another place and you can fly there, just by leaping off the rooftop and finding your flight.

The waterfall drops off into another place you cannot see.

It is where you can begin to teach yourself how to journey within your mind.

You can imagine anything you want...anything at all.

You can see beyond the reality of Earth and look at your inner universe with creativity and imagination.

You can picture a rainbow bridge to fly over that will lead you to another part of your kingdom.

You can picture a flying Pegasus who will transport you wherever you want to go.

Here, in your kingdom, there are no rules.

You are the one who decides how your world will look and how you will find your way forward...

Enjoy flying over your inner kingdom, and let keep unfolding for you.

Breathe steadily.

You can land anywhere you want and take off anywhere you want.

You are flying in order to get a bigger picture, greater scope and nothing is too big or too small here.

It is everything you ask it to be.

[Give plenty of time for creative visualization and meditation here]

Your world is an awakening place.

It helps you find your creative life-force, your deeper truth, your secret purpose.

This world within your mind is a sacred landscape, a dimension of your thoughts and your feelings, to be explored like a great adventurer seeking hidden treasure in every cave, forest, and hideaway...

Bringing your focus back to your breath.

Let yourself continue exploring in ways you may not have before.

Let yourself delve more deeply into these ascended places.

Who do you meet along the way?

Have you met another spirit guide or ascended master who comes to teach you a lesson of healing and spiritual wisdom?

Do you have any specific places that you feel more draw to in this unique universe?

Wherever you are in your flight, give yourself a moment to see if you can find your castle again from this point of view.

Can you tell where you are on the map of your mind?

Are there secret tunnels and portals that will lead you right back to your castle?

Begin to find your way back to the castle now, breathing steadily and slowly along the way.

You can see it, and it feels far, but you have the ability to fly.

It won't take long to get there.

You are feeling more peaceful now and ready to fall fast asleep.

Your journey through the kingdom has shown you much and given you mush to appreciate.

You follow your original path back to the mirror where you first began.

Down, down, down the stone steps of the castle, like you are unwinding...

As you come to the mirror again, you see your eyes again, your face, your body.

You see your outfit.

It may have changed, and that's okay.

Or perhaps, after flying through your inner world, you are ready to take on a new form.

How do you want to dress now, as you prepare for a wholesome night of gentle, peaceful rest?

What would feel best to you right now after feeling the freedom of flight?

Take a few moments and breaths to see yourself in the castle mirror...

Now, you are ready.

You can now retire in your inner kingdom, in the castle of your dreams and imagination.

Exercise

Core Belief: --

Evidence supporting belief: Evidence contradicting belief:

----------------------------   --------------------------

----------------------------   --------------------------

----------------------------   --------------------------

----------------------------   --------------------------

Chapter 33. Water For The Queen

There once was a young knight named Pip, and Pip admired his queen. The Queen of Alanstar was one of the fairest women in the land. She had a mature demeanor, but creamy white skin, and long-flowing, silky black hair that seemed to envelop her throne. After the King passed many moons ago, the Queen ruled the land with a fair amount of care.

One day, the Queen summoned Pip to her throne room. The young knight bowed to his queen.

"What do you desire?" he asked.

"Good afternoon, my dear knight. I'm currently low on drinking water, and the knights who normally bring it to me are taking the day off."

Pip scratched his head a bit. There was plenty of water around. But before he could ask, the Queen answered for him.

"I drink the water from the peak of the Wellspring Mountain. At its tip, the cleanest, clearest water known to man resides. They say a fairy lives on top of the mountain, purifying the water. As it goes down the mountain, it becomes a little less pure, but still drinkable. However, I desire only the cleanest water the land has to offer. Could you give me a pail of it?"

Pip nodded. All his work for the Queen so far had been to mop up the castle, or to change her bed covers. This was something that maybe, just maybe, she'd reward him with.

The Queen handed him an empty pail, complete with a lid. This golden pail had some jewels in its rims, and it looked a little tacky, but shimmered, nonetheless. Pip immediately set forth after some preparations. He put everything on his trusted steed, Pap. Pap was a beautiful white horse who served him well in the few years he had been a night. With Pap by his side, Pip told him to giddy-up, and they were off, away from the castle's stables and to the unknown.

The Wellspring Mountain was not too far from the Kingdom of Alanstar. Its water, minerals, and wildlife all nourished the kingdom quite well. With that said, there was still a bit of travel before he made it to the kingdom, so Pip trotted down the field, seeing all the sights.

And so, their journey up the Wellspring Mountain began. The sound of the stream brought some relief, calming Pip's racing mind. Despite the climb, this task seemed safe. The scariest threat Pip faced so far was black bear that lapped up some water out of the mountain, but that bear just looked at Pip and paid no mind.

The water seemed to have a calming effect towards nature, and Pip and Pap stopped a few times to taste the mountain's water. It was already so clear, clean, and tasty. The Queen must have been really picky about her water.

Despite the initial climb being a bit of a breeze, the mountain soon began to steepen. There was a point where Pap made a sad whiney, unable to go any further. Pip hopped off.

"You just stay here," he said to Pap. "And I'll handle the rest."

He tied Pap next to a stream, leaving some oats behind. Pip unloaded any unneeded gear he had expect for his mountain climb, keeping only the pail, his equipment needed to climb, and the corn that Pop gave him. It was a long piece of corn, and quite filling. He munched on a bit as he began his climb up.

Pip's heart beat a bit as he climbed up, going higher and higher, and his axe sinking into the mountainside. The cool, fall day soon became one that was a bit chillier the higher he went. The cool breeze danced around his temple and made his teeth chatter a bit, but he continued to climb.

As he climbed, with only his thoughts to entertain him, his mind began wandering. He was a kid again, training with his friends, their swords connecting in a rhythm that made him smile as he thought about it some more.

At the time, both him and his friend, Jaq, who since had departed for the Kingdom of Pio, always declared their love for the queen. "I'll be the queen's bodyguard!" Pip declared.

"No, I will," Jaq countered, and they continued to fight.

Pip chuckled as he climbed onward. He guessed this fight was still going on, even if Jaq had long since left the kingdom.

Pip continued his ascent, the temperature growing a bit colder and colder but he still persevered. He could see his skin reddening, and a bit of snot ran down his nose, but he still climbed. The queen would love him for this; he just knew it!

After what seemed like an eternity, he could see the top. Pip climbed straight to the top, and there, at the apex of the mountain, he saw something that made his eyes widen.

It was a beautiful hot spring. Steam rose from it, the heat immediately ridding himself of any potential frostbite he may have had. So, these were the legendary hot springs where the kingdom got his water. Here, the water was at its purest. It was hot, but free from any dirt, toxins, and packed filled with minerals needed to keep the body going.

Pip filled up his own canteen with some of the spring water, as he'd try it himself. Then, he began filling up the pail with the water. Soon, the pail was filled up, and he screwed the lid on. The water was safe and secure, and the way down was always better than the way up. Pip was about to make his way down, when he realized something.

This was probably going to be a once in a lifetime opportunity. Why couldn't he relax a bit? Pip took off his clothes and hopped into the hot springs. The water was that perfect balance of hot, but not too scalding. He felt the minerals kiss his skin, and the steam cleanse him of anything dirty he had on it. He let himself drift off a bit, almost falling asleep at the mercy of the springs. Ah.

"Hey!"

Pip opened his eyes. In front of him, a woman the size of a ruler floated above him, translucent wings flapping. She had crystal blue eyes, hair the color of a mountain snow, and a frown on her face.

"I spent all the time purifying the water, and yet, here is a man who dares to dirty himself in the springs. You should be ashamed of yourself."

Pip rubbed his eyes. Maybe he was just seeing things, but in front of him was a

"Fairy!" he exclaimed. He stood up and hopped out, and the fairy fluttered to where he was.

"Of course," the fairy said. "I am the Great Pixie, and I clean up all the water. But the water won't be too clean if you contaminate it. It's going to take me hours to purify it again! You should be ashamed of yourself. I ought to turn you into a mountain toad!"

Pip gasped. "I'm sorry," was all he could mutter. "I've traveled for so long, just to fetch a pail for my queen, and I wanted to take a break."

The Great Pixie nodded. "I don't blame you, but don't do it again. Gee, though. Fetching a pail for your queen? That sounds like a whole lot of work. Is she paying you well?"

Come to think of it, Pip shook his head. "She gives me payments for cleaning her room and for doing tasks, but it's just enough to eat and nothing more."

"Then why do you do it?" the pixie asked.

Pip scratched his chin. "I do it because I love my queen."

"Yeesh," the Pixie uttered, fluttering around Pip as she shook her head. "You do realize that she isn't going to 'return the favor,' if you get what I mean, just because you did something nice for her."

"Buzz off," Pip said. "I know what I'm doing."

The Pixie shook her head again. "Men, I swear. I'm glad I'm a pixie and not one of you humans. Anyway, I suppose you should be going. Go serve your queen or whatever."

Pip opened his eyes. He was back taking a dip in the hot springs. As he stood up, he looked for all signs of the pixie. However, she was gone.

"Did I fall asleep?" he muttered. It seemed so real. The fluttering of the wings, the sassy attitude, it all seemed to happen not too long ago in a plane that resembled reality. And yet, here he was, just a fool who almost drowned in the hot springs.

With that, he put his clothes back on, grabbed his pail and canteen, and began the journey down. As expected, it was a cakewalk. He sipped from the canteen when he was about halfway down. It tasted crystal clear and as he drank it, it felt like the water was washing everything unclean from his body until what was left was a crystal-clear interior.

Pip soon reached the bottom, and there, he met Pap again and began his journey back to the kingdom. The sun began to set as he made his way to the castle. Soon, he was back at the throne room.

"I see you are back," the Queen said. "I thought you may have fallen off." She chuckled a bit as he laid the pail at her feet. She opened the pail and sipped from it.

Pip smiled. "So, my lady, what do I get for doing all that work for you?"

The queen tapped her foot. "Well, our budget is a bit low, but I'll try to compensate you soon. Otherwise, your work here is done."

Pip sighed. "Is there anything else you could give me?"

Exercise

Alternative belief:
_____
_____
_____
_____
_____

Chapter 34. The Old Woman

Darlene was a forty-something-year-old woman who had spent her entire life doing everything that she knew she was supposed to do.

She woke up every morning at six to feed her dogs and her cat, she made breakfast for her children and her husband, and she fixed a pot of morning coffee. When everyone was fed, she would clean their plate's away, tidy up the kitchen, and help everyone get ready for their day. Then, it was off to school.

Darlene would then head into the office to work until the school day was over. She would then go pick up her children, bring them home, feed them a snack, and escort them to their after-school activities like soccer, dance, and swim lessons.

When everyone got home in the evening, Darlene would fix up a supper, feed everyone, and then clean all of the dishes when everyone was done eating. She would then clean up everyone's bags and shoes, tidy up any other messes that had been made that day, and then sit down to watch thirty minutes of television before bed.

On weekends, Darlene would do all of the same things except instead of going to school or work she would take her kids shopping, to sleepovers, or to their sports events. There was always something going on, and Darlene was always in charge of having to make sure that everything got done in time.

When she was in her early forties, Darlene realized that she was entirely miserable. After spending nearly two decades cleaning up after her family, preparing meals for them, and driving them around everywhere, Darlene realized that she was done.

She no longer cared to have the experience of doing everything herself, as it was beginning to take a toll on her. She found that every morning she would wake up depressed and dreading the day before her, and every night she would go to sleep sad and wishing that she could wake up to a brand-new life. This brought Darlene great guilt as she loved her family and loved caring for them, though she could no longer do it all by herself.

One day, Darlene was called into her boss's office in the middle of the afternoon. As she got up from her desk and headed toward her bosses office, Darlene tried to recall anything she may have done wrong that could result in her being talked to or written up by her boss.

Of course, she could not think of anything she had done wrong as Darlene was always very particular about doing everything properly. After all, she was great at doing what she knew was expected of her. When she reached her bosses office, Darlene's boss asked her to sit and offered to get her a beverage.

Darlene agreed and began sipping on the tea that her boss had brought her as she tried to understand what it was that she had been called in for. To her surprised, Darlene's boss offered her a promotion that came with a substantial raise and increased benefits compared to what she was already receiving.

Darlene was excited by the offer, but at the same time, she was miserable to realize that taking it meant that she would be committing to staying in this lackluster life that she was no longer getting joy from.

Before she knew what, she was doing, Darlene refused the promotion and instead put in her notice and quit her job. She went and cleared out her desk and left, never to look back again.

Darlene's family was surprised to learn that she had quit her job and had no intentions of going back. They were also surprised when she said that she would no longer make breakfast unless she felt like it, that everyone would need to find their own ways to their hangouts, and that the only thing Darlene would help with anymore was getting to sports events or homework.

At this point, her kids were old enough that they could walk, bike, or even drive themselves to their own events so she would no longer have to do it. In other words, Darlene was ready to start letting her children grow up and become young adults.

Asserting these boundaries meant that Darlene had great freedom in her life to do whatever it was that she pleased. She could sleep in, eat whenever she wanted, and even watch afternoon television shows that she had heard her friends talking about at the PTA meetings at her children's school for years.

Finally, Darlene got what it meant to slow down and just be, rather than to always have to be in motion doing everything in her power to please everyone else.

At first, Darlene's laid-back lifestyle was enjoyable as it offered her a great change of pace from what she was used to. Over time, however, it grew boring as she realized that she would always be doing nothing unless she did something to change that. As she did not want to spend her entire life bored, Darlene began looking into different hobbies and discovering new things that she liked.

One hobby she found that she was drawn to was making jewelry. Darlene found that not only did she enjoy making jewelry, but also that she was incredibly good at it, and that people often wanted to purchase her jewelry.

Darlene started out making jewelry as a hobby in the afternoons while she watched daytime television. She would make four or five new pieces per week, and inevitably every single piece would sell to someone that she knew.

Eventually, she started selling her jewelry online as this gave her the opportunity to sell even more.

Before she knew it, Darlene was making copious amounts of jewelry and selling them to friends, family, strangers online, and even stocking it in boutique stores around her town. She grew so excited to make jewelry that Darlene would excitedly get up in the middle of the night and sketch out new plans, or launch from bed in the morning ready to start crafting new creations.

Although it was a far cry from what she was used to, Darlene loved her new life of making and selling handmade jewelry.

Her children and husband liked it as well, as they began to realize that Darlene was happier and enjoying life once again. It took them some time to get used to Darlene not being available to help as often anymore, but in the end, they were all happy that Darlene had found her passion and that she was finally enjoying life after helping her family do the very same thing for so many years.

Exercise

When you're ready to face your fears, here are ways to get started:

1. Complete a CBT diagram of your fears, identifying your relevant thoughts, feelings, and behaviors and their relationships.
2. Look for subtle ways that fear affects you that aren't immediately apparent.
3. Choose strategies from the Think, Act, and be categories to practice in the coming days.
4. If you have specific fears that lend themselves well to exposure therapy, begin with step 1 and work consistently through the plan.
5. Balance the tough work of facing your fear with consistent self-care. Being good to yourself will help you through this process.

Chapter 35. Dandelion Wish

The summer was as gorgeous as any Jenny had known.

Days of running through the sprinklers, and going out to the lake, and having picnics in the local park.

Roasting marshmallows in the fire pit out in the backyard, making s' mores, and enjoying family get-togethers around the barbecue.

The weather was warm but cold lemonade and shade under the trees helped to keep everyone cool.

Jenny worked hard and brought about many changes: remodeling the home, taking on a new role at work, helping her daughter recover from her very first exciting school year.

Tonight, Jenny sat with Kirsty out by the fire pit in the fading evening light.

The others had gone inside, but she wanted to spend the night with her daughter and enjoy one of the last nights of summer.

The smell of wood smoke drifted on the air. Gentle pops and crackles accompanied the embers that floated up in the air, glimmered, and went out.

One of Jenny's favorite things in the whole world was to sit next to a fire and enjoy the warmth and flickering glow, and the sound, the smell, all of it. She loved it, and now she had passed that down to her daughter, as well.

The steady sound of crickets and the occasional hoot of a night bird made a relaxing chorus to lull their heavy eyelids ever down further.

"I want a story, Mom," said Kirsty, yawning heavily in her chair. Then she hugged the blanket she had brought outside even closer around her.

Her head leaned back, but she was not ready yet. Jenny had brought out a sleeping bag because sometimes they liked to sleep out under the stars, on perfect nights like tonight.

Kirsty got out of her chair, went over to the sleeping bag, and slid into it, the fabric swishing loudly as she snuggled in.

Jenny moved her chair over near the sleeping bag.

"I thought you might, honey, so I came prepared!"

"How are you going to read in the dark, Mommy?"

The flickering firelight did not offer much steady light for reading, but Jenny only smiled.

Jaina ran barefoot through the dandelion fields.

Soft grass and cold, moist dandelions comforted her feet as she ran, springing up again as she passed through.

Other flowers stood amid the dandelions but she loved them all equally. There were white flowers and pink and blue ones, all set against the deepest green grass, and the dandelions shone like droplets fallen from the sun on high.

The smell was so divine! Aromatic grass, wild and thick, met with the fragrances of sweet nectar.

Breathing it in was like feeling the soft petals gently caressing her face. Jaina could never get tired of it.

She knelt down and scooped a fuzzy white dandelion out of the earth. Holding it aloft, some of the seeds began to blow away on the wind.

Jaina watched them float, and she laughed because that was exactly what she wanted to wish for.

"I wish I could fly as you do, and see what you see!"

Then she pursed her lips and blew, scattering all but one seed from the dandelion head.

Countless flowers waved in the breeze, each a little point of light, like a star in a deep emerald sky. About they wove beautiful music, thousands upon thousands of voices raised up together in song.

The wind whooshed and the dandelion seed soared as the ground fell away in rolling hills. She lifted higher into the sky, where winds flowed like river currents in an invisible ocean.

The sky darkened. Something passed by overhead, giving out a proud cry.

It was an eagle, soaring with its feathers in the sun. Jaina beamed as she looked up at it.

She had always loved birds, admired their freedom in flight, and now she has to experience the same thing.

The dandelion seed caught an updraft and higher she went still, hot on the tail of the mighty eagle.

Floating beside it, she laughed, and tears streamed from her face, in sheer joy.

This was something she had always wanted, and now her wish had come true!

Trees rose like spires from the land, each holding an entire world in their branches.

The eagle saw all: the scurrying squirrels and the nesting birds, the hares and the deer, the fish gleaming in the far-away streams winding about the feet of the trees.

Here, this place was alive with the fullness of the summer, an inexhaustible flame of vitality.

Beyond the green and growing things, the eagle saw the spirits of land and sky, which frolicked as happily as a bird on the wing.

They were tiny like Jaina, or big like the eagle, sometimes both at once. Their lives mirrored that of the land itself.

Where they trod, life bloomed, and where life bloomed, they gravitated, forever finding meaning in the growth of the smallest seed, or the tranquility of the tallest tree.

Jaina realized that even during the day, when most were wide-awake and stretching out beneath the sun, the world dreamed, and she floated through its dreams at once an observer and a fellow traveler.

She breathed in deeply as the wind rushed across her face, granting her a sense of freedom she had never know before.

Here, sailing upon the sky itself, she knew what the golden days of late summer meant to all that lived within them.

She could feel the vibrant pulse of the world hot in her veins. It gave her such a sense of purpose, an invigoration that nothing else could match.

"You must not forget this feeling," said the eagle.

"This is life, my friend. Life at its purest. Enjoying sun, star, and moon. Breathing in the wind. Flying freely. You could weigh as much as a tree and still not burden me, for I am free. Here you are free, too."

A rocky outcropping stood tall over the bank of a wide blue lake below.

The eagle dipped his head. "Farewell, friend! Return whenever it pleases you!"

Jaina dove from the eagle's head turned and waved goodbye to him as she fell.

She spread her arms and let the wind slip through her fingers, cool and soft.

The lake grew as she fell toward it, but she was not afraid. Like a drop of rain, she broke the surface and plunged into another world.

The lake welcomed her as it welcomed the sunlight, which cast rays that soon became swirling mist within the waves.

And in the water's cold, refreshing embrace she saw more travelers. Big, silvery fish, their eyes bigger than her sprite-sized body, swam past, lazily enjoying the warm waters.

Jaina found that she could move through the water as freely as the eagle had the air, and she glided over to a bed of kelp that grew outward like a swaying forest.

A soft song like a hum rose from the kelp, celebrating its perspective: a green plant that enjoyed both water and sun in equal measure.

Jaina reached out and touched one of the leafy stalks and for a moment saw what the kelp saw: an entire kingdom stretching out across the bottom of the lake, and a sky ever shimmering at the surface.

Fish hid within its leafy mass. Crawdads crawled across the silt within its reach. Frogs and tadpoles danced to its endless tune. Ducks in the water sent ripples ringing like notes across the wave-sky above.

Pieces of driftwood floated by and some of the kelp would seize onto it, pulled free to drift with the wood.

The kelp saw all these lives bound together by the water and the growing earth and the sweet air above. Its perspective was truly blessed, to know so much of the lake's grand symphony.

Jaina swam back to the surface, buoyed by the haze of sunlight filtering down through the water.

She surfaced, listening to the plink and splash of the water.

Jaina lay back and closed her eyes, floating like a flower petal and simply enjoying the relaxing sounds.

She slept, or perhaps sleeping was the same as waking here, where dream and reality were one.

When she opened her eyes, no time had passed at all. The sun was still high in the sky above the lake, and a warmth rippled across the water.

Her breathing coincided with the rise and fall of the gentle waves. In, the water rose, lifting her toward the sky. Out, the water sank, and she felt cradled in a cool liquid bed.

In. Out. A year could have rolled past and she was so calm she would have never noticed it.

Presently a deep hum beat the air. Jaina opened her eyes.

A dragonfly hovered over the lake surface nearby, landing on a small piece of driftwood.

To the rest of the world, it was only a few inches long, but to Jaina the traveler, it looked to be closer in size to an actual dragon!

"Hello!" she called, waving. The dragonfly turned its head to her and its wings buzzed.

"Hello. Fine day, is it not?"

"Yes, it is!" Jaina clapped, incredibly amused that the dragonfly had answered her. "I have never enjoyed the lake so much."

The dragonfly buzzed in agreement. "Oh yes. The sun is pleasant and the water is refreshing. But I must be going. Will you need a lift?"

Jaina's eyes lit up.

Jaina looked down at the lake slowly strolling past beneath her, an amazing view of its shimmering surface from high up.

Never before had she had such a perfect wish granted?

A white cloud descended to fly next to her—no, not a cloud, the dandelion seed.

Exercise

Keep in mind that the goal is not to banish anger from our lives. Instead, we can learn to keep it in check.

1. Complete a diagram for a specific situation that made you angry to learn more about your own experience of anger.
2. Use a thought record to capture and examine some of your anger-related thoughts for a situation that comes up.
3. Begin to note situations in which you'd like to practice managing your anger.
4. Choose one or two techniques from the Think, Act, and be categories to start practicing.
5. Write down how each technique works for you, and add new ones as needed.
6. Refer to your list of strategies often to remind yourself of the best ways for you to manage your anger.

Chapter 36. Beneath The Waves

Jane plunged into the water, feeling the unwieldy weight of her diving equipment leave her instantly. The water lifted the burden from her back and, as she adjusted to the breathing apparatus, her attention was placed squarely on herself.

Finally adjusting to the pressure, the shifting presence of the tank on her back, the pressure of her diving suit, and the pressure of the goggles on her face, she was able to look around at the stunning world around her.

She could see the other divers from her group plunging into the water around her, taking pictures with their waterproof cameras, taking in the wildlife that skittered and flowed beneath and around them, and marveling at this whole world that lay beneath the island where they had been vacationing.

Jane floated for a moment, looking into the deepening expanse that lay before her. As she stared into the distance, she could see the shimmering blue of the ocean darkening toward the horizon.

She didn't expect to be able to see so far ahead of her or that the water would look so calm from underneath the surface. She could see fish lazily ambling through the water, barely taking heed of, yet relying on the currents in it.

She made her way closer to the white sands that lay at the bottom of the ocean. The water wasn't terribly deep here, so she knew she could swim down to it without getting lost or putting herself out of her depth.

In the white sand, she saw many small shells and sensed a movement that came from the current that danced above. As she watched the sands arrhythmically moving, she saw a small crab pop up from beneath the surface and scuttle under a nearby rock.

She gawked at the life that teemed around her, swimming from place to place and admiring its beauty. As she did so, she found herself drifting further and further away from the boat that had brought them to the diving site. They were told they could go pretty far away from the site, but to stay close enough that you could still see at least one other diver.

She made sure she could see one diver as she continued looking for more pretty sights to see under the waves. As she hovered in the water, she swore she saw something whip across the floor beneath her. Slightly alarmed, but trying to keep her breathing even, she looked around to see if she could find the thing that had slipped past her.

Over the occasional hiss of her breathing apparatus, she heard the gentle swish of quick motion through the water behind her. She whipped her head around, but still heard nothing. Out of a sense of fear and self-preservation, Jane made her way back over to the group. She stayed with them until the session was over and uneventfully made her way back up onto the boat.

In her hotel room, she couldn't help but think about the presence that whipped around her in the water. She really had seen it there, right? It hadn't been some figment brought about by the heat from being on the beach all morning before her dive, had it? Either way, she needed to get back to the water to figure out what it was.

She looked out at the ocean from the balcony of her hotel room. She could see the spot where they had been diving that day. It was dark out, so there wasn't much of anything to see in that spot. The waves on the water were choppier than they had been in the afternoon and the wind had kicked up slightly.

She felt compelled to watch that spot in the ocean as the wind blew and the waves rolled. She was unable to take her eyes off the spot where they had been that afternoon, and he had also been unable to figure out how she knew that was where they had been. She hadn't even needed to think about it; she just knew that was the spot. As she pondered this, eyes transfixed on that spot, she saw something glowing beneath the surface. Something... big

She wanted to call the front desk and ask about the thing glowing in the ocean, but she couldn't bring herself to move from that spot. From the muscles in her forehead, all the way down to her pinky toes, she could not compel any muscle in her body to move even the slightest bit, as it would mean possibly interrupting her view of the brilliant light that blazed beneath the waves. She could swear, as she watched it, that it was getting brighter and larger at a pace that her eyes could barely process. It was slow but certain.

Her ears twitched as she watched the light. Was it... Singing? It sounded like a hum, a screech, a hymn, and a bell, all rolled into one song. It was not a cacophonous sound, though her mind seemed to insist that it ought to have been for all the elements that it contained. She was thankful that she couldn't will herself to move. Everything in her mind was screaming at her to jump over the railing of her balcony and into the ocean to see what was calling to her from the deep.

Before she could make heads or tails of all the things that were going on at that moment, everything went dark. The song, the ocean, the light, the room, the city below... Everything, All at once, the waves in the ocean completely subsided and settled into a calm, glassy surface that reflected the moon, which somehow also seemed muted. She felt the tension in her muscles release suddenly and before she could compensate, she tumbled to the floor, losing consciousness on the way down.

She awoke the next morning to the sun shining through the open balcony door, birds calling, and calm waves crashing periodically on the beach below. She was still on the floor, wearing her clothes from the evening before. She picked herself up off the floor and made herself take a shower, get some coffee, and get dressed. Once she had taken care of herself, she would get some answers about what had been going on the night before.

She entered the lobby and saw that it was business as usual for the guests and employees in the resort. People were milling about, asking questions about gratuities, breakfast, check-in times, and scheduled tours. She peered around to see if she found anyone that looked anywhere near as unsettled as she felt but there didn't seem to be anyone who fit that description.

She walked up to the concierge desk to talk to the sharply dressed woman there that wore a bright, happy smile.

"Excuse me," she started.

"Yes, madam; how can I be of service?"

"Do you know anything about the blackout that happened last night? What was it that caused it?"

"I'm sorry? Did you lose power in your room last night? I can ask the front desk if there were any interruptions they might know about."

"No, I mean the blackout in the whole… Did the city not lose power last night?"

"No, ma'am, I don't think there was anything like that here last night. Would you like me to ask the front desk?" Jane's mind was racing.

"Oh… No, that's okay. Thank you." Jane didn't wait for a response before she went back into the elevator and ran back up to her room. She changed into her swimsuit and ran back downstairs and out to the beach.

She asked about scuba tours that would be going back out to that spot, but the instructor said that there wouldn't be any tours that day due to a family emergency for the instructor. The man at the booth was simply there for equipment rental.

She rented the equipment she needed and suited up, heading right for the spot where she had been diving the day before. The spot where she had seen that impossibly large light, how had no one seen it? How had no one reported on anything that had happened the night before? Had she suffered some sort of heat exhaustion that made her imagine the entire thing? Maybe this solo vacation had been a mistake after all.

Once she was certain she had all her gear on properly, she dove into the water off the platform that jutted out into the water. She looked around for any sign of the presence that she had felt the day before. At first, there wasn't anything strange going on in the water around her. In the silent calm of the water, she began to feel silly. Maybe she had just chased a complete illusion all the way out here and maybe there never was anything strange in the water at all.

She turned around to make her way back toward the ladder that extended into the water from the platform off of which she had jumped. As she swam toward the ladder, she heard it. Her blood ran cold and she felt the hot tingle of alarm pulse through her body. She stopped swimming and listened for a moment. When she heard nothing further, she turned very slowly to look at what had made the noise.

Nothing, before she could feel anything at all about the lack of a presence in the water with her, she saw it. Something barreling through the water from leagues away, it was impossibly swift; ignoring any resistance the water should have posed. As it dashed toward her, it kept its eyes fixed on her.

Her muscles once again refused to move in any measure as she met its eyes. Dear Lord, she thought. It's massive.

Its eyes seemed miles wide as its gaze held hers. In seconds, the monstrosity covered an incredible distance. Jane tried to brace herself for impact as it closed in, but she could only float, powerless. Its immense mouth opened as it got mere feet from her. Its teeth were jagged and craggy. Each one would have been deadly on its own if it had been wielded by a person. Lined into the gaping maw before her, they were the gateway to oblivion.

As the darkness enveloped her, she could swear that she heard humming... Humming that also seemed like a screech, a hymn, with just a hint of bells. My God, it's beautiful, she thought.

Exercise

If you're ready to take advantage of the many benefits of exercise, follow the steps

1. Start by defining what's important to you about physical activity. For example, is it about doing something that brings you joy or feeling like you're taking care of yourself?
2. Find activities you enjoy, which may not even fall under the label "exercise." They might include going for walks with a friend, playing tennis, or taking a dance class, for example. The more you enjoy the movement, the more motivated you'll be to do it consistently.
3. Plan specific times to exercise, and schedule them in your calendar. Start gradually so you won't feel overwhelmed by your goals.

Chapter 37. All I Have Got

Stepping out of the kitchen with a dish of breaded pork tenderloin sandwich, Mrs. Simpson headed straight for the dining table, but was interrupted by a beep from the desktop computer, which lay in one corner of the sitting room. She rarely uses the computer except when she had important emails to attend. However, the computer was a constant companion to Derrick, a 12-year old boy who happens to be the only child of the Simpsons. Since Derrick traveled to Hills town for holiday, the computer was rarely used. Mrs. Simpson had put the computer earlier to reply to some emails. Mrs. Simpson resisted the urge of going over to the computer; she instead went to the dining room and served dinner for her and her husband.

Your cooking skills haven't deteriorated at all remarked Mr. Simpson as he gulped down the last drop of water in his glass cup. He was fond of teasing and complimenting his wife at any slightest opportunity. If there was a perfect couple, they were one good example. Everything seems to be working perfectly fine and it looked as if they were special and specifically meant for each other. Blessed with good jobs, a good house, and a son, what else could they have asked of? While Mr. Simpson worked as an accountant for an auditing firm, Mrs. Simpson was a high school teacher. Both loved their profession with passion and would often debate on which is more important to society. Such debates would always end in Derrick averring that the pilot is the best profession. He had always dreamed about being a pilot.

Mrs. Simpson's attention was drawn to beep she heard from the computer as she went to sit on the sofa in the sitting room. She quickly went over to the computer and hit the enter key. To her utter consternation, the mail she received sapped the life out of her. Her husband's contract had been terminated with immediate effect. Before long, tears rolled down her cheeks, her world came crumbling down around her. Though she has a high school teacher, her husband provided the majority of the finance for the home. How would she break this sad news to her husband when he comes out of the bathroom?

Although the air conditioner was working efficiently, it wasn't enough to cool down the temperature of the house. Mrs. Simpson had broken the sad news to her husband in the early hours of the following morning. It was indeed heartbreaking information that he never wanted to accept. He went over to the computer for personal verification. His wife wasn't wrong after all, with a rubric written in bold red letters it read 'LETTER OF CONTRACT TERMINATION'.

Mr. Simpson could hardly believe his eyes, what had he done wrong? Did he breach the terms of the contract? Millions of thoughts raced through his mind, he sat simply dumbfounded and dejected. Determined to prove to himself he didn't properly understand the content of the mail or the company made a mistake, he picked up his phone from the table and dialed the company's number. His fear was confirmed; he had been sacked as the company retrenched staff. The recent development took him miles off his pace and he decided to go on a stroll with his pet.

The school was three days away from resumption and Derrick had to come back from holidays to continue his studies. He was expected back home on Friday evening and his mother made his favorite meal. The day seemed longer than usual for Mrs. Simpson who hadn't set eyes on her son for over two months and was very anxious to see him again.

The Simpsons were getting very worried; it was already 7:53 p.m. the manager of Fantasy World Park had earlier told them Derrick had boarded a bus back home. He should have been home by now muttered Mrs. Simpson. Though her husband was worried, he didn't make it visible. At about 8:48 p.m. Mrs. Simpson received a call from an unknown caller. She was always skeptical about picking calls from strange callers, but in this case, it seemed she was anxiously waiting for the call. Regardless of the fact it came from an unknown caller, she swiftly picked the call.

Oh no! Oh no! Were the only audible words Mrs. Simpson could stutter over the phone? It was yet heartbreaking news. Derrick had been involved in a ghastly accident and he lost his life. A young boy full of potentially losing his life just like that, how tragic! Mr. Simpson had always been a strong-willed man, but in this case, he couldn't withhold the drops of tears as they streamed down slowly down his cheeks. Here he was, losing two very important things in his life within the space of days. First his treasured job, now his one and only precious son.

Life hasn't dealt fairly with me at all he said amidst sobs of deep contrition as his son was laid to rest. It was indeed moments of sadness and grief for the Simpsons. Having lost his job, Mr. Simpson decided they move to an affordable apartment down the street. Though they moved physically, their fortunes skewed negatively. Things went from bad to worse and you could hardly tell this was the same happy family who had everything going for them a few months ago. Well, in all honesty, life isn't fair after all.

Despite moving to a more affordable apartment, the Simpsons still found it difficult to foot the bills. They were neck-deep in debts, electricity bills, water bills and other bills just piled up like ahead of sand. As the days rolled by so did the debts. They were literally living from hand to mouth with little or nothing to show for their endless day and nights of toil. Determined to salvage their dilapidating situation, Mr. Simpson suggested they get a loan from his former employee. This suggestion was met with utmost enthusiasm and sigh of huge relief by his wife who saw this as an opportunity to start afresh, make a new beginning.

As they walked past the traffic light in the cool of the evening, Mrs. Simpson noticed a figure that looked familiar. On closer examination, it was Duke, one of her students in high school. What are you doing out here all alone by this time of the day questions Mrs. Simpson? Duke was dumbfounded and could barely muster a reply. Following several persuasions from Mrs. Simpson, he finally laid out his predicaments. 'Ma, I lost my parents a week ago and I have absolutely nowhere to run to, no apartment, no food, no clothes, nothing! Please ma, help me'. These words resonated in the mind of Mrs. Simpson who had compassion for the boy. However, Mr. Simpson was indifferent and couldn't wait to leave that place and head home. He had also faced his own fair share of life challenges and he believes everyone should be able to bear his or her own cross.

You can't do that Mr. Simpson cut in as he jolted back to his senses from his wild thoughts about life. Mrs. Simpson was about rendering some financial assistance to her students from the loan they had earlier secured. This decision simply didn't go down well with her husband and he stormed off angrily seeing his wife remained adamant about helping the boy. Damn! I can't continue living like this he said to himself as he boarded a taxi and zoomed off.

Well, said Mrs. Simpson, I actually wanted to give you a part of this money to help you, but this is all I've got. Take it, make good use of it and one day when you assume a position to help others, and don't hesitate to do so nonetheless. Mrs. Simpson ended her short sermon by handing over the entire funds meant for offsetting some of their debts and starting afresh to Duke. This is all I've got she reiterated, please manage it. Full of thanks, Duke knelt to show appreciation, but Mrs. Simpson urged him to get up and ensure he makes judicious use of the funds made available to him. Duke thanked her for some more as she went on her way.

On getting back home, Mrs. Simpson noticed her husband wasn't at home. Mr. Simpson arrived very late at night and complained bitterly of his inability to carry on. He requested a divorce, but his wife turned it down. Mr. Simpson seems to vanish into thin air as he hasn't been seen since leaving the house the following morning. She tried reaching him on phone severally all to no avail. For over a few days she made frantic efforts searching for her husband. Although she was hindered by her apparent lack of financial resources.

Exercise

Ready to put your plans into action? You can start with these steps; focus initially on the ones that are most important to you:

1. Take stock of whether you treat yourself like someone you care about. In what ways would you like to treat yourself better?
2. Plan and start a consistent routine that prioritizes your sleep.
3. Make one positive change in your nutrition plan—for example, preparing a certain number of meals at home each week.
4. Add more movement into your day. Start slowly and build gradually.
5. Create a stress-management plan; include one small daily activity (e.g., listening to relaxing music on the way home), one bigger weekly activity (e.g., taking a yoga class), and one monthly activity (e.g., getting a professional massage).
6. Incorporate more time in nature into your week: combine time outside with social contact if possible.

7. Look for small ways to serve others every day, as well as bigger service projects to do on a regular basis (e.g., volunteering weekly at a food bank).
8. Write down three things you're grateful for every evening before you go to bed.

Chapter 38. The Rookie Detective

It was a hot, lazy afternoon, and all I had on my schedule was tackling the bulk of paperwork littered on my work desk. I tagged a pile of papers "Overdue" and another collection "Terribly Overdue," in hopes that the tags would propel me to do the needed work. It wasn't working; however, I cared more about the large chunk of pizza that sat right in front of me. I've always been terrible at paperwork, and some 10 years back I thought paper documentation would be extinct by now, but here I was with so many papers to sort and very little field involvement to prove myself. I was desperate for a chance to unravel tough, mysterious cases.

"I can do this! I have to!" I picked up the "Terribly Overdue" bunch of papers, unbound them and made to work when my phone buzzed, taking me off balance. The caller ID flashed across the screen.

"Detective Mike Powel"

It was quite unlikely for him to call me. I know it can't be for good. Two minutes of tense conversation ensued over the phone. After this, the papers were hastily arranged in an order no one else would understand and crammed into a filing cabinet. The keys to the patrol car were lying somewhere under a stack of files and it took some ransacking to find it. I dashed out of the office, then came back for two massive bites of pizza and guzzled some water, it was now warm from direct sun rays, but I couldn't care less.

Having spent all day indoors and staring at papers, my eyes squinted in the bright sun. "Okay! Here we go. It promises to be a long day" The tires screeched as I made a sharp turn out the parking lot and off to the road. The road wavered before me as I sped along the highway on full throttle. If Detective Powel's voice over the phone was anything to go by, it meant I needed to be there in real-time. I wasn't about to pass up on the opportunity to get some rare field involvement.

As I stepped out of the car, lots of cameras, recorders, and microphones rushed towards me with an avalanche of questions from the reporters. "What's your comment on the situation?" was one of the numerous questions I could pick out, probably because most of the reporters practically yelled that at me.

"No Comments," I said as I stepped over the ribbon that barricaded the crime scene. It was an elementary school building, although all students and teachers have been evacuated. As I stepped into the room, I caught a glimpse of Detective Powel's gloomy face. He had a profound love for kids, and with four adopted kids in his custody, you could imagine how much the body bag that laid on the floor tore him apart. From the shape and size of the bag, I could tell it contained a child below ten.

I dived into the work of investigating what had led to the death of the child with all the strength I could muster and started rummaging through the bulk of papers when something caught my attention. It was a case file for a child that mysteriously died some three weeks back. I was to compile it and send to Chief McCourt. Flipping through the pages revealed that he died in the course of the night. There was no sign of struggle, no fingerprints were found in his room. CCTV footage in the neighborhood didn't reveal anything relevant to the case, although there was no

CCTV installed in the home of the deceased. "How can this be?"

Those pages marked the end of my paperwork for the night as I pondered over them, going through over and over in a bid to comb out every piece of information, and maybe find out something no one had found out. The boy died without any form of struggle. No fingerprints were seen in the areas. No footprints. And you know what's worse? It's the second time Taggart is experiencing a similar occurrence in three weeks." I made no headway until I woke up lying on the sofa in my sitting room.

I always wake up very early in the morning. Today, it took the timely intervention of my fiancée, Alissa, to get me off the bed. I could be late yet again to work, I hurriedly took my bath and dashed off to the parking lot where my black sedan was parked. I quickly zoomed off into the ever-busy expressway and made for work. Though she has often complained about my complete immersion in my work, I sincerely wished she really understood my predicaments. I was way too preoccupied amongst other things with the huge pile of paperwork which seems to multiply as the days' rolls by and the case I had been assigned to.

It was yet another day at the CTPD, officers adorn in their custom uniforms walked frantically to and fro. On my way to my office, I walked past Detective Scott and greeted him with a grin on my face. I never bothered whether he responded or not. Detective Scott has been quite pissed off since I was given the mandate to handle the recent case of the death of an elementary school kid. The vibe I had on entering the CTPD main building was almost sapped completely on sighting the huge pile of papers I had to attend to on my desk.

In particular, one caught my attention; it was lying reverse on top of the pile. On closer examination, I discovered it was a circular from Detective Powel. For a brief second, my heart skipped a bit. He rarely sends circulars to my office. What have I done wrong? I said to myself as a quickly glanced through the contents of the paper. On the circular carried the instruction that all detectives are to meet at the intelligence room by 9:00 a.m. I sought to complete some of my paper works before heading to the intelligence room.

On entering the intelligence room, all the seats in the front had been occupied. Obviously, I was the last detective to arrive. Detective Powel gave me a disapproving look as I quickly rushed to assume a seat at the back of the room. Detective Powel was known for his short, but in-depth briefings. Today was quite different, he seemed a little bit uneasy, unlike his usual calm self. As he put on the projector by one corner of the room, several gruesome images of a young boy about thirteen years old displayed on the big white screen in front of the room. It was indeed a very tragic picture to behold, what could be the cause of this? I wondered. Again Detective Powel cast a very long gaze at me and said: "You are in charge of this case, I want situation report and update every 24 hours." Although this came as a surprise and rare privilege to me considering I was already working on a recent death case, I was very much disheartened for the deaths of those innocent persons at least before proving otherwise.

I got hold of the relevant documents and information I needed to kick start the investigation. On getting back to my office, I decided to have a closer look at the case files. Here I was, a rookie detective with very little prior experience of actual field investigation saddled with the responsibility of two death cases in quick succession. I quickly perused the files and made for the scene where the incident occurred.

Completely perturbed, I laid out all the papers and images handed over to me by Detective Powel. I stared at the papers that lay before me like a chess player contemplating his checkmate move. The longer I stared, the more exhausted and frustrated I became. I never noticed the presence of Detective Scott, just as he caught my attention. He smiled and with a pat on my back he said, "You always wanted a case to investigate, congratulations now you've got one." As he walked out of my office, I was caught between getting angry with his statement or motivated to get to the bottom of the case. The latter was my choice and I sincerely hoped I have no regrets whatsoever in the future.

After staring at the papers lying in front of me for a few more minutes, I decided to take a much-needed break. I headed out of the CTPD building and went across the street to one of my favorite spots. Though it was a café, I personally took it as a relaxation spot and unwinding center. As I ordered for my favorite soft drink, I briefly glanced at the 43" TV which hung delicately on the wall. News from the TV filtered through the sound waves in the café, but unfortunately, none really interested me. It was the usual day to day stuff about government I always heard, but most importantly I couldn't afford to add any of the news headlines to my current to-decipher list.

Just as I sipped the last drops of the soda drink from my glass, I overheard a news of two missing school children. Suddenly, the news I despised a few moments ago completely stole my attention. I listened carefully as the newscaster read out the details of the missing schoolchildren. The children had gone missing four days ago here in Taggart. This was the second time this week I heard a news about school children missing without any trace. I felt compassion for the children and most especially their parents who will be worried sick of their children. I thought over the missing children for a while, but quickly had to remind myself I had enough tasks on my hands that needed urgent attention. I paid for the drink I ordered and customarily left a tip for the waiter.

I went back to my office and the rest of the day was uneventful. I spent most of the time staring at the papers lying on my desk in the exact spot I left them with hopes that the answers would just pop up. I resigned to taking all the case files back home. Though this was unethical, some of the detectives had to do it in other to fast track their investigations. Just maybe Alissa who is a lawyer could help me trace and link the disjointed lines. Going back home today, I wasn't particularly happy. Here I was as a detective unable to make any headway and coupled with the missing children, I could barely think straight.

Exercise

For this, consider the following questions:

- What is the number one issue you hope this exercise will help you with?
- What have you tried so far to get some relief?
- What has worked well and what hasn't?
- How does CBT as I've described it compare with what you've tried in the past?
- Finally, how are you feeling after reading?

You need a journal that's dedicated to your CBT work. If you don't have one already, plan to get one before you start

Chapter 39. Wet Dreams

My buzz is back and not just from the marijuana. Dalton's cock looks like the high dive from this angle.

Laying on my back, I can wink at the ceiling cam as my hot boy toy strokes himself with his eyes burning holes in my tits. I'm amazed he's so enamored with the girls. No doubt, I'll have fun with this one with my hubby. Having a nineteen year young ogling my thirty-eight year old tits is better than getting carded buying alcohol.

"Wanna titty fuck me?"

Dalton flinches then grins like Lucifer. Without saying a word, his lubed up cock (he used up most of my Vaseline on that diving board) is sliding between my boobs. I press them together. The hair on his balls tickles me as he humps my humps. His cock bangs into my chin—I swear that beast keeps growing.

Dalton's eyes squint and his face contorts.

"Cum on my tits."

The first spurt drills my chin then he unloads all over my tits. After he's spent (for at least a moment), I say, "That's fucking hot. Nobody's ever cum on my tits before."

Dalton chuckles as he says, "I'm your first." His eyes dart away from the mess he leaves on me as he grabs my phone. Snapping a pic, he says, "We gotta send this to your husband."

I feel triumphant for influencing Dalton to play along with our fucked up fantasy.

Dalton takes a swig from his beer bottle. I say, "Hold that bottle next to your cock once."

"Why?"

"Another photo op. Hand me my cell."

Dalton says, "We should take the pic with me hard, don't you think?"

"I want a before-and-after. Besides, your flaccid cock is bigger than most guys' boners."

I aim my cell as spunk trickles down my belly. And before I can take my before pic, my stallion is hard again. Most guys enjoy me saying they have a big cock, but Dalton loves it. He holds the bottle beside his statue schlong and, just as I thought, he's as thick as a bottle.

"Does my talking about your big cock excite you?"

"I was thinking about fucking you doggy style actually."

"Oh my God Dalton, you've already blown five loads. Where do you get the energy?"

"I can't get enough of you and your tight wet pussy. Hey, can I tape me fucking you doggy style?"

I grin at the cell, then say, "Do you want to fuck me like an animal?"

"Yessss," Dalton growls.

I prop myself up on all fours and wink at the teddy cam, then turn and lock eyes with Dalton and say, "Fuck me doggy style naughty boy!"

Dalton lunges behind me and his cock tip grazes my ass. "Wrong hole, go lower."

"Oh sorry."

"Do you want to fuck my ass?"

"I dunno, maybe..."

"Maybe? You're the first guy who hasn't begged to fuck my ass. For your tenth orgasm, I'll let you fuck my ass, but put that big cock in my pussy for now."

I gasp as his cock enters (my pussy). From this angle—and given how wet I am—he slides in so fast and far, I fear he'll puncture my lung. His balls slap my clit so I know he's all in.

He's sliding in and out in long slow strokes that stretch my pussy walls to the max. I wince each time his balls slap my button but manage to keep my eyes on the teddy cam. I say, "You're cock is so hard."

"Does this hurt?"

"Yes, go slow, I'm not used to such a big cock." I lick my lips for the teddy cam.

"Can I film this now? I want to remember this moment forever."

"Dalton, that's so sexy..."

"So I can then?"

"Ok, as long as you don't get my face in it...and promise to jack off to it when you get home."

He pauses and my pussy gets a welcome momentary break as he grabs his cell off the night stand. I hear a click but don't turn around—fearing my face would end up all over the net. But my fear is overcome by the fact that he wants to video a woman twice his age. He has no idea how much he turns me on. It's as if we feed off each other's energy in a perpetual state of libido.

He resumes fucking me from behind slowly. "Talk dirty for the video," I blurt.

"Check this out. I'm fucking a MILF doggy style...look at that great ass."

As much as I like being associated with MILF and great ass, I hope he puts the cell down soon and focuses on fucking me. He sounds like he's filming a freaking documentary. I yell, "Fuck me harder."

He pauses again and I hear his cell clank on the table. I turn and corner-eye him as I say, "Is this better than you imagined when you jacked off?"

"Hell yeah!"

"Then fuck me hard."

I look straight ahead as Dalton rocks my body with his powerful thrusts. He's teasing my G-Spot and the pain from before is pure pleasure now. I reach down with one hand and tweak my pearl.

Dalton moans as he short strokes deep inside me.

And before I can explode, Dalton is already spurting.

I'm not complaining. Please don't get me wrong. Turning on a guy half my age is the equivalent of an orgasm. Ok, not quite, but eventually, he's going to last long enough for my volcano to erupt.

For a moment, I consider pulling my vibrator out, but don't want to completely freak him out. In a way, coming so close to cumming stokes my libido like never before. Mike always makes me cum before he unloads. But I can't remember the last time Mike came twice in one night. Dalton is already on number six of what will easily hit double-digits soon. Hell, at this rate, he'll shatter his orgasm record before midnight.

Believe it or not, I miss Mike right now. I wouldn't trade him—even for Dalton. Well, maybe for one night, but not every other night.

Dalton reaches for his last joint and all I want to do is soak in the tub. yourself.

Exercise

The top five positive qualities and values I want to cultivate in my most important relationships:

1. --

    1   2   3   4   5

2. --

    1   2   3   4   5

3. --

    1   2   3   4   5

4. --

    1   2   3   4   5

5. --

    1   2   3   4   5

Chapter 40. Spanish Trip

During this trip to Barcelona, I want to treat myself to a front-row seat at a Flamenco dancer's performance. I've heard amazing stories of passion, emotion, and the energy of their art form, and want to experience it for myself.

To begin my evening, I start in the early afternoon on an outdoor patio with some tapas and two glasses of vermut, the unofficial beverage of Barcelona. The small bites are delicious and make excellent use of the region's offerings of fresh seafood and the most perfectly ripe tomatoes I've ever enjoyed. Vermut is an inexpensive yet delectable wine. It is enhanced with cinnamon and cloves, and I pick up hints of chamomile and rose. It warms me, and I leave the street pub with my appetite primed as I hear toward the gothic quarter for a slow walk to my show.

In the oldest part of the city, the sun begins to set the fading light casts long and interesting shadows across the landmarks. I remind myself to keep moving, to not get drawn in by the texture and the details of every new building I pass by in this labyrinth. Most of these streets are closed off to traffic, and I am free to roam as I wish, zigzagging from one magnetic feature to the next. Through one narrow road, I pass under a footbridge high above my head. It is decorated with details, the masonry of the arch at its base, and the latticework under the railings. The piece that genuinely catches my eye is the lace-like stonework that floats between the columns and arches along the top. I stop and marvel at how it was possible to create such a delicate work of art out of something as unyielding as stone. I sense I am not the only viewer and notice a couple has stopped and joined me in admiration of the architecture. "Beautiful, isn't it?" the woman remarks, to which he replies, "not as beautiful you, my love." They share a tight embrace and carry on with their sunset tour of the gothic quarter.

My walk carries me to the doorstep of the Barcelona Cathedral, the home of the Archbishop of Barcelona, Catalonia, Spain. It was on a previous trip that I discovered the long, rich history of the Catalonian people and their lifelong fight for the right to be an autonomous province. One of only four in Europe that lasted throughout the ages. It is an honor the people of Barcelona do not take lightly. This cathedral is dedicated to a patron saint of Barcelona, a young woman who suffered martyrdom at the hands of the Romans. The cathedral built in her honor soars over the old city, and its pointed spires still gleam with the last rays of sun sinking into the Mediterranean. The nested archway pointed bell towers, and dozens of gargoyles that dot each available point create a castle-like resting place for the spirit of the young woman.

I reach the hall of the Flamenco performance and hear the musicians from inside, easing the audience into the ambiance with the harmony of four guitars, the gentle drumming of Cajon, and the unmistakable clacking of castanets. The soothing strum of classical Spanish guitar draws me in, and I find my seat at the front of the stage just as the lights dim to signify the beginning of the dance. The music slows, a tall woman in a long, ruffled black dress emerges from behind a curtain. She walks to the middle of the stage; her look is serious. Her stride is purposeful, and at center stage, she assertively stomps both feet. She turns to the musicians, raises her arms slowly and delicately above her head in a fluid motion, a dance of their own.

The entire room holds their breath in anticipation. In a flurry of movement, melody, and a touch of madness, the musicians strike up their song. The dancer claps along in a feverish rhythm and tells a story through her body. I am entranced by her power and elegance, the speed and precision that she maneuvers her feet, and hands and emotions in time with the music. She directs the musicians, challenging them to keep up with her creativity. She is the matador and the musicians her bull, her body is the cape, and they are all entwined in the organic masterpiece of Flamenco dance. I lose myself entirely in the moment as each enters and exits the stage, each with a story to dance and a passion for sharing. An hour after the first chord is strung, I find myself in a standing ovation, clapping vigorously with the rest of the audience in total awe of what we collectively witnessed.

The show is over, and audience members pour out of the hall and into the dark streets of Barcelona. As I walk, I try to mimic the skill of the dancers expressing themselves in dance. I gain an immediate appreciation for just how challenging the art form is. I hear laughter behind me and turn to see I am not the only traveler to make an attempt. We share a smile about our shared clumsiness, and I begin to walk back to the hotel. I pass by a small restaurant, with its table still out on the patio, and I recognize the couple from our bridge earlier in the evening. She is sitting on his lap, and they share a delicious looking dessert, he feeds her a bite, but it falls onto her skirt, they laugh. I hope they jump up and perform a dance to illustrate their innocent and passionate love for each other right there in the street.

Exercise

Feeling Identification

Exercise time: 10 minutes

Benefit: Identifies and expresses feelings

MATERIALS: Paint pens, crayons, or markers (whichever you prefer); 1 sheet of 18-by-24-inch heavy-weight drawing paper

1.   Choose a color that reflects how you're feeling today.

2.   Draw a circle with that color.

3.   In that circle, use lines and shapes to draw an image or images to identify how you're feeling today.

4.   Name your art.

Chapter 41. The Writer

Norman Alderman was a single man of the age of 48. Each and every new day, he worried more about being single. It was 2012, and all of his friends, by this time, had children, and some of them even had grandchildren. But then he thought, "I guess I shouldn't worry about that because we are all different now, aren't we?" Norman was taken to standing in front of the mirror, seeing himself as a playwright or famous novelist receiving a Pulitzer for his magnificent work. What Norman saw in that mirror was Charlton Heston. What the mirror showed was Woody Allen. He did have one redeeming feature, though; he was smart. At least he thought he was smart. "Aren't all people like me smart?" he mused.

Norman was a writer. He thought he had what it takes. Actually, that's not true. He was trained to be an accountant. He had worked in that field for six years and saw himself as a tiny little man at a tiny little desk in a huge office full of tiny little people. He did not like that view, so every day, he went home and meditated. While in his meditative state, he tried to make himself wake up a famous and successful writer, but every time he pulled out of it, he was still a silly little ineffectual, Jewish man. "Well, at least I'm good at meditating," he thought.

Norman was a persistent man, although, at times, he wondered what he should do with his free time, should he quit writing and do something else. "No," he thought, "that would be giving up, and I'm not a quitter. I'm not," he repeated to himself in his mind. "I write, therefore I am a writer!" he exclaimed to himself. "Who am I talking to?" he asked, hoping nobody else ever heard these musings should they think of him as wonky. So, Norman wrote. He wrote poems, short stories, and articles. He had files of pieces that he had written. All of them good, but all of them good enough. "If I can just get that winning piece, that one literary achievement." He muttered. "If I could just do it?" Each evening when he went to bed, he saw himself as a great writer; he just knew he had it in him. If it would only come out

It was Friday afternoon, and he had just got home from work at his accounting job. He thought about calling his friend, who was also an accountant and who also wore horn-rimmed glasses, like him, but she wasn't a writer. She was a real accountant. In fact, she was the boss's number one bean counter. "I think the boss is a little like me, a little lonely. That's probably why he likes her?" he questioned in his mind.

One thing that you should know about Norman is that he is eccentric. He loved his computer and owned an old tower that he just kept fixing. He also owned a laptop, but he wrote on neither of these machines. He had inherited an old Remington Rand from a family estate, and he felt that the machine gave his writing work character. In fact, he felt that the old machine gave him character.

That night, Norman had an idea. He scrambled over to his typewriter, dropped into his seat, and placed a brand-new blank sheet of typing paper in the machine. "Let's see now," he said. "What can we call this piece? I know," he said excitedly. "We'll call it the writer!" He placed his palms facing outwards, interlocked his fingers, and pushed out cracking all of his knuckles at the same time. Then he placed his hands in the writing position on the typewriter keyboard. When he began to type, something magical happened. It was as though his fingers were doing the thinking. they flew over the keys getting far ahead of his mind. How can this be, he asked?

He looked up at the clock. "Wait a minute now?" He said. "I know that the clock is at twenty after four because I just looked at it a minute ago. Now it says 6:30? This is amazing," he said, "but it can't be?" he thought. "I just work for 2 hours? There must be some missing time somewhere." But when he looked down at what he had written, he skidded his chair back wildly and tore the paper from the typewriter. "Did I write that? I wrote this! I did it! I do have the touch!" Then, realizing that the piece was only just begun, he replaced the paper in return and sat down again to continue. A small amount of drool emanated from the right corner of his lips. He didn't notice this. He was so deeply involved in what was happening. He felt a strange power overtaking him. At first, he thought, "Well, this is not right?" but then he said, "The heck with that! This is me! This is me doing what I do best. I am the writer!"

Norman typed and typed! He typed on that old Remington until midnight and then typed some more. He wasn't even looking over the script that he was writing; he did no "on the fly" proofreading at all. This wasn't like him. He usually took more time staring at what he had written than doing the writing itself, and this gave him thought. At 2 AM, he stopped. His writing was scaring him.

At one point, before sliding the chair back from the desk, he thought, "this is just wrong! I like being in control of me." But when he read over what his crazed fingers had written, all that went out the window. Why he had written about himself, or at least that's what he thought at first. But when he got into the piece, he noticed that the man's name was Chad. "That's not me?" he said to himself. Then he read the entire piece and began to write more.

Chad was an attorney but had never won a single case. The state put him in charge of handling the defendants who couldn't afford to hire their own attorney. He was a "Court Appointed Lawyer" and a loser. The problem was that his heart wasn't into it. He wondered how he could have picked the wrong career. He wanted to be a writer, so every night, he wrote. "The small and fruitless man sat down at his computer and began to write. He wrote and wrote until his fingers were tired, and his brain was on fire. The story took the form of a woman by the name of Edna, who was a writer, and had no confidence, but kept on writing day after day anyway, and did finally produce something she liked.

At first, Edna thought that she was writing about herself, but then she noticed that she had typed a name. The character was called Joyce, and Joyce was a winner. She entered contests and won them. She didn't know why, and she had no plan that could possibly be called a system, she just won. Why just last week, Edna wrote, Joyce had won a brand-new car. It was just a little front-wheel-drive Ford with a tiny little engine that sat sideways in the front. Joyce was happy with it though although Edna wrote, she was worried that she would have to pay some sort of tax on her new car value when April rolled around again. The following month, Edna wrote about Joyce again and decided that Joyce, would enter the Readers Digest Sweepstakes. Of course, she won the big prize, which was no surprise to Edna as that was all in the script as the saying goes. Edna wrote that Joyce was overjoyed but not surprised and she won half a million dollars and just put it in the bank, and kept on living the same way as if nothing great had happened.

Norman loved his coffee, and sometimes on the weekends, he would take his laptop and sit in the local coffee shop drinking coffee and writing. It was a Saturday morning, and he decided that this would be one of those days. He packed up his trusty old laptop and headed out. When Norman arrived at the coffee shop, he realized it was still very early, and the place was nearly empty. "Where shall we sit this morning?" he asked himself. "Ah, the table in the back, that's where we'll park it." He sat down and plugged in his computer and then went up and ordered his coffee and a pastry.

He cracked his knuckles the way he always did before he started to write, and then returned to his work in progress. The story about the writer named Chad. He wrote for a long time and didn't notice that the shop had become very crowded. A woman had taken the seat across the table from him but way down at the other end, and then a young man came in the shop with his laptop and looked around. He noticed the empty seat next to Norman and walked over. "Do you mind if I sit here and work?" he asked Norman. "Be my guest," Norman said without looking up from his screen. He heard the man shuffling around and plugging in his machine but paid no heed. He was a writer, and he must write.

Then Chad suddenly sneezed, and Norman said, "Gesundheit." "Thank you," the young man said. "Are you a writer?" the man asked and then, "I'm sorry, may I introduce myself, my name is Chad." The man said. Norman's head jerked up in surprise. After typing the name Chad over and over for the last month or so, he was shocked to suddenly meet a man with the same name. He noticed that Chad was holding his hand out and waiting to shake Norman's hand in their meeting. "Uh, oh sorry," Norman said, "I'm Norman, and yes, I am a writer." "Me too," Chad told him.

"Now this was starting to be very freaky, Norman thought. Could there be this kind of coincidence?" he wondered. They both returned to their respective laptops, and another half hour passed. Then Chad got up and went into the restroom and left his computer open. Norman thought, "Oh no, you don't? That would be very disrespectful. After all, you wouldn't want anyone looking over your shoulder trying to see what you were writing." But he couldn't control his curiosity, and he knew that was a weakness. He looked. He saw the word Edna and almost jumped out of his skin. He looked again and noticed that in Chad's story, Edna was also a writer. "This just can't be!" he thought in a panic.

Exercise

Prioritize items on the list. By indicating which items are high priority, you can be sure to do those ones first and can relax about not getting to the lower-priority items right away.

Ready to make your own to-do list using these principles? You can use the template below to write down activities you need to complete, including their due date. Then give each task a priority level (e.g., low/medium/high, or 0–10). Finally, schedule a time in your calendar to complete each activity.

PRIORITY   TASKS   DUE DATE

Chapter 42. Mark

Every time Mark placed his hand against the bottle of beer, and he felt the coldness of it, something tingled in his being. From the back of his head, through his spine, and ending in the middle of his butt. That had been the only refreshing experience that he had known for the past three months since Lizzy left him. Shocked? Yeah, he was shocked that Lizzy could leave. Yet had he expected it. The warning signs had come, they were flashing in his eyes. At least he could not deny that one. She was unaffectionate, she could not be satisfied, and she increased the tempo of her nagging, hell, he could even say by a hundred percent. It was all just unexplainable, and he wished things would get better. Just like most stories like this, they never did. So, he just waited for what would unavoidably come, Lizzy, leaving him alone in the darkness that had consumed his soul with the prolonged times of strive and the likes. This is why there could be no other thing that he could rely on than on this fragile bottle, which he knew would one day send him crashing to the floor. Why he kept on to that too, no one could tell.

"When are you going to quit?" Clark asked him.

"I don't know, man. I just don't know," Mark replied.

That was the most real person he had still, but he walked away. Clark could not tell of any way he could have helped Mark. Any light that was truly going to set him at liberty would have to come from deep within himself.

"Help me, Lord," Mark muttered more often than ever.

On this evening, he had said the same words, while he yet turned to the green bottles at a bar. But on this evening, he could not deny, there had been a great restlessness over his being, all over. There was nothing he felt that he could do about it, but he knew the way to his favorite bar, and that was just where he went. If the universe ever did its work, or say, something like destiny, that must have been what was at work that evening. He met Tom, a lazy folk that walked into the bar. He had taken a couple of beers and seemed terrified. Frantic, he began searching all over for where his purse had been. He looked so much in panic, that Mark's attention, even in his depression had just been drawn to him. Mark was halfway through his drunkenness. At this stage, he could still comprehend to an extent of decent reasoning, but the speaking part was not so much what he could put up with.

"You little runt, you had better bring out my money or I am squeezing you till there is no life in you," the angry barman had said.

Why was he being so unfair? Could he not see that the little man had truly lost his wallet, and who knows what with it?

"I swear to you, man, I swear to you, I do not know where my wallet is. It was just here right now, right here with me. I swear it. I think I have been robbed!" Tom yelled, enough for every person who had been in that bar to hear him loud and clear.

"Every thief swears he is not a thief. I stole my wife's money last night. I swore on my mama's grave I had not even been at home at the time she speculated," a drunken man yelled from another side of the bar.

His comment was accompanied by the laughter of others. The barman did not seem to enjoy the rowdiness of the bar, but he had his eyes stuck to the little thief. Mark took his time to examine him for the first time. He seemed a teenage or a little above it. Say he was twenty-one or twenty-two.

"I can swear I have heard of this kind of trick before. You drink and you don't pay and you fake the loss of your wallet. Fucking loser. You are going to pay every dime or you will lose bones in your body tonight. I swear that to you," the barman said, sounding angrier. He had been a really big man, even he seemed larger than the regular size. At this point, he seemed to be advancing towards Mark, and there was no smile on his face.

"Leave him alone, I will pay," Mark said in his drunken tone.

"What?" the barman and Tom echoed together in unbelief.

"I will pay for the lad. Let him be. Add his bills to mine," Mark repeated, as he pushed a wad of cash towards the barman.

"Thank you, sir," Tom said, shyly, towards Mark.

"You're welcome," Mark mouthed at Tom.

"You lucky beast, now get out of my bar," the barman said, angrily.

As Tom tried to get himself together, preparing to scamper out of the bar, Mark spoke again.

"Nah! Let the lad stay with me. Let him drink as much as he wants to. The bill is on me," Mark said.

Tom looked at the barman and gave a sheepish smile. Furious, the barman slammed a rolled towel against the slab and walked away. Tom, at this point, made fresh orders from the other barman and he sipped slowly and gracefully. There had been silence between them, in what seemed to be like through the entire bar. Tom passed cursory looks towards Mark and wished he could do something, or better still, say something to make him know that he was grateful for what he had done. Mark saved him the stress by speaking first.

"You did not have a wallet, did you?" Mark asked.

"Sir?" Tom pretended not to have heard the question.

"I did silly things like that as a kid too, you know." Mark continued.

"I am sorry sir, but sometimes, it just gets also crazy that a guy needs more beer than he can afford, you know?" Tom replied.

"Were those not the things that made us light enough to think we literally floated through life, being weighed down by nothing?" Mark asked.

Tom turned to examine Mark for a moment as though he could not believe the things that he was saying.

"Exactly sir, exactly," Tom finally replied.

They continued drinking and did so for a short while.

"You seem like the married kind, are you?" Tom asked.

"Is that a pleasant way of saying that I look stressed?" Mark asked, laughing.

"Perhaps," Tom replied.

"Well, I am not married," Mark said.

"Then what brings you here, why do you want to float?" Tom asked.

"Escape," Mark replied.

"What from, if I may ask?" Tom askes.

Tom went wordless for a short while. Meticulously, he took sips at his glass.

"Boy, I was once like you, you know, free and flying. Then I met this woman that I know I truly loved. Then things began to fly high for me," Mark began to explain.

He put his hand in the air, like a bird and he glided from the point of the table to higher and higher.

"Then all of a sudden, dash! I crash down like a little bird," Mark concluded.

"What struck you in the air, truly?" Tom asked.

"What do you mean? I just told you a woman I loved left me and that affected me so bad. What do you mean what struck me, kid?" Mark asked.

"Most times, we know what happens to us, but what we do not investigate is how we let what happened to us, really happen to us," Tom said.

Mark dropped his glass and looked into his eyes in unbelief.

"I swear, I have never heard a drunken man so wise," Mark said, laughing.

Tom burst out in laughter too and soon, they were both laughing out loud.

"Tell me though, what struck you. How did you give in?" Tom asked again.

"You know, it was obvious we were headed to that direction of things, but I kept hoping, holding on, something like that. You know. I kept wishing, even though I knew all was gone. Maybe that was not the crime," Mark replied.

"What was the real crime then?" Tom asked.

"Waiting to be loved, not knowing I had the power to love myself," Mark replied as he raised the glass again to his lips.

Tom gave no response to what he had said. He seemed melancholic, his face reddened after a while.

"What is wrong with you, man?" Mark asked.

"I remember when my mama died. Every single evening, for two months, I walked up to her grave to weep. I looked at the gravestone, looked at her picture in it and just cried. It was a festival of sorrow, every single day for sixty days or more," Tom explained.

"Oh, I am sorry about that," Mark replied.

"Then one day, I come to realize that I was drilling through the same sore that I hoped would heal. I discovered that deep down I did not want it to heal, I wanted to feel the pain over and over again. I thought that was the best way to keep alive her memory in me. I thought it was love, but I got to the realization that love was more. Love meant keeping ourselves strong too, and not feeling the worst for those we loved. Love meant letting go too. Then I chose to let go. It took a while, but I let go in the end," Tom explained.

Mark was silent.

"This is no philosophical shit, man. I mean it from the depth of my being, man. Let go. Walk by, walk past. That is life. We walk by things and people, if they are not meant to be with us, we must learn to walk past," Tom said.

"I hear you, kid," Mark replied, sober.

"Holding on to the blade that cut us would stitch no wound, man," Tom said.

In Mark's mind, he knew that it was true, everything that Tom said to him.

"I want you to go home, get yourself together, and be the best of you that you can be. All of this is for yourself. You have tried so long in being the best for others; you must put in the same energy for yourself now," Tom continued.

Mark thought about everything that Tom had said to him in that instance. He observed Tom as he hurriedly gulped down what was left of his beer mug, then he stood up to go.

"I have got to go, man," Tom said.

"But why, there is still much more to drink," Mark said, surprised.

"Perhaps. But I drink to enjoy and not to die. I have got no worries to drown," Tom said, patting Mark on the back as he walked away.

Mark wished after Tom had walked away, that he had gotten his phone number. Talking to someone of that kind.

Exercise

Begin by thinking of one particularly important person in your life and the relationship you have with them. Write down all the good qualities you like in this person.

- This exercise has to be interactive, you are allowed to consult.
- The exercise should not run beyond 20 minutes

Chapter 43. The Dimensional Life Coach

Charli and Pam were happily married and were going out tonight. It was their anniversary, and they were still just as much in love and infatuated with each other as the day that they met. They were two very lucky people, as they had learned over the years that many of the people they knew from their college days had also married but were now divorced. This, they attributed to the fact that they had always meditated together since the beginning, and that meant that they were two very relaxed people. They were, however, looking for something new to do and decided to take a trip to Hawaii.

They flew over to Oahu and stayed in a rental overlooking the Ala Wai. One night, they went out to a Luau. Neither of them had ever been to one before, and they had a blast together. They stayed all the way until the end and then decided to take a walk. They went back to their rental car and got a pair of flashlights they had seen in the trunk. The party was on the beach but far down the coast and away from the main part of town. The beach was bordered by a deep and lush forest of Hawaiian foliage.

They looked at each other and shrugged their shoulders. "Why not?" they thought as they entered the dark canopy.

They didn't get far before they fell upon a huge rock face with a cave in the bottom of it.

Again, they looked at each other and said, "Let's check it out." Turning on their flashlights, they entered the cave, and after walking only a few feet, they sensed something happening to them.

Looking down at their hands and feet, they noticed a vibration, and everything was becoming a blur. Then a blinding flash of light and they were in a long swirling and twisting tunnel. Bright colors were flashing all around, and they floated freely but were turning head over heels and had no sense of gravity.

Then it was over, and they were standing on a grassy knoll near a river, but something was very wrong, and they both knew it. The grass was green, all right, but the river was orange.

Charly thought that he knew what had happened, and he explained it to Pam. "I have read about this stuff," he told her. "I think we may have stumbled on a portal to another dimension. They say there are many dimensions, and in each one, there is another you and another me doing something very different than we are doing in our normal dimension."

Pam listened.

"So, in this dimension, you may have tried to do something that you love like perhaps play the piano with hopes of being in an orchestra. But you found that you were not good at the piano, so quickly dropped that dream. But in another dimension, the same you may be a critically acclaimed pianist traveling the world and very famous." Charly finished.

Charly knew that if this was the case if they had been sucked through a portal, that they would need to remember where it was so they could return to their dimension, or they would be stuck in this world forever. He made some mental notes about the exact spot they landed and which direction they were facing when they landed. Then, they decided to explore. They would follow the orange river to see where it took them. It flowed lazily past them with a bright and luminescent orange glow. They followed it down the hill for a little way and came upon some animals. They were the size of rabbits and seemed to have the same demeanor, but their fur was bright red. They had huge bright blue eyes that looked like crystals, and they stared at the couple as they walked past.

Then, they arrived at the bottom of the hill where the river dove under a long winding road. It didn't look like a traffic road like we were accustomed to seeing but had some sort of strange metallic tracks that wove back and forth over each other.

"What sort of crazy train could fit on those tracks?" Charly asked to himself.

They crossed the unusual looking road and noticed a slight grade now going uphill again. They trudged up the hill, and when they reached the top, they both had their breath taken away for what they saw far below.

It was a massive city structure with towering pointed buildings that glowed in reds, blues, and yellow hues. It was as though the buildings themselves were radiating the light rather than being lit up by another light source as they were accustomed to in their home dimension. They saw that down at the foot of the buildings, there were waterways, and the orange river that they had followed down earlier must have been flowing down to the city.

There were also odd-looking flying crafts going in and out of the buildings at all levels. Just then, they heard a scuffling sound behind them as though somebody was walking past. They turned just in time to see a creature that was about four feet tall that had stopped and was standing and staring at them in the same way that they were now staring at it.

"Greetings, friends!" a voice said.

Charly and Pam quickly looked at each other. They had both heard the voice, and they had both been looking at the little being when they heard it, but its mouth didn't move at all.

Charly thought he knew why that was and stilled his mind. "We are visitors to your land and mean you no harm," he thought, believing that what they had heard was a telepathic communication.

"Yes, that is fine. How did you get here, and what is your name?" the voice came through again. Charly held his hands slightly out and up with the palms facing up in a gesture of friendship and took several cautious steps forwards towards the being.

"My name is Charly, and this is my wife Pam," he said, gesturing to where Pam was standing.

"Ah, good." The little being said, "we are establishing mutual communication and seeking common ground between us. I am Remicon Whaler, and it is fine to call me "Remi." It said.

Then, Charly dropped his arms and gestured to Pam to walk with him towards the being. As they got closer, they noticed that its eyes were reptilian and yellow with black vertical slits for the iris. His skin was a deep purple color and had a luminescence to it that shone the light in other colors when he moved. They saw a beautiful deep turquoise and a dark crimson that glimmered from every part of his skin. He was not wearing any clothes but looked very natural. He and no hair, and they noticed that he had large gills in the sides of his neck. Overall, he was actually quite attractive to the eyes.

"Remi, can you tell us where we are because this place is not our home. We were on vacation in Hawaii and went exploring in the jungle. We had not gone far before we were sucked into what appeared to be a wormhole or some kind of time gate. And now we are here in this beautiful place." Charly said.

"Yes, this is our home, and it is quite nice, isn't it?" Remi said. "You clearly entered by mistake, and I know how to get you back over to your dimension. You see, we here live in a closely guarded dimension, just one shift away from yours. We often use the gate you found to enter your world, but generally, there are no visitors like you ever come here. It is intriguing that you were able to do it." Remi told them.

Then Pam spoke up. "Remi, do you mind if we ask you some questions? And you, of course, can ask us as many as you like as well but we are curious. What race lives here, and are you a part of that race?" She inquired.

"Oh yes, of course, you would want to know more than just where you are, wouldn't you?" Remi mused.

"Why don't we all go to my home. It's not far from here. Would you like that?" he asked.

Remi led the way down a path we had not noticed until it came to a meadow. The path had been closely bordered by some sort of jungle plants that were about 5 to 6 feet high, and the meadow was absolutely stunning. We saw large blue trees that all had twin trunks. I don't mean that they split like our trees do, but rather came out of the ground as two separate trunks. The blue color gradually became a dark purple as it reached to heights above the meadow. The canopy was bright orange and seemed to intensify the sun's rays as they shone through it to reach us here down on the ground. And the flowers! We saw reds, blues, pinks, and white flowers everywhere. This place was much more beautiful than our home dimension, and Pam and I were amazed and impressed by it all.

"Here we are," Remi announced as we came upon what first appeared as a wall of blue wood-like substance. As I followed it up, I noticed it was actually a massive tree. The thing was so large that you could only barely determine the gradual roundness of the huge trunk. It was gargantuan. As we followed Remi towards it, a large door materialized, and we stopped before it.

Remi made an odd gesture with one of his hands, and the door opened sliding straight up. "Welcome to my home friends," Remi said as we all went inside.

Pam and I tried to cease appearing, amazed at everything when we saw the lush interior of Remi's house. I will just tell you that if the meadow was amazing, Remi's home was beyond that by many degrees. It was like walking into a massive aircraft hangar, which was furnished with Ethan Allen type furniture.

"Would you like tea?" Remi offered.

"That would be lovely," Pam responded. We both sat on a bright red soft bottom couch that must have been 25 feet long, and when we did, a recliner-like footrest seemed to come out of nowhere, and our feet were gently cradled.

"Here we go," Remi said, placing three cups of tea on the small table in front of the couch. "Please, ask your questions now." He said

Exercise

Begin by closing your eyes and imaging a peaceful world with no hurt or pain. This exrcise should be able to help be calm and happy before bed.

- This exercise has to be interactive, you are allowed to share the experience with your partner.

- The exercise should not run beyond 20 minutes

Chapter 44. The Stairway Between Realms

In the fabric of space and time, there is woven a passage that allows for travel between. The realms were not knit as a waterproof cloak. There are seams and streams that beings can slip between. A displacement of creatures in the wrong time or a displacement of matter in the wrong space is a hint at this "Stairway between Realms." It has been used by the bold and brave to pass to new dimensions and discover new secrets. Many geniuses have wielded this power to expand their minds. But there is a danger there.

If you travel for too long along the Stairway Between Realms, you may lose your way. The passage is not clear as a hallway or a literal stream. It was a convoluted maze that intertwines and intersects upon itself. Imagine an ouroboros that was eating its own tail, but twisting and knotting itself as it did so. This is what the Stairway between Realms can be like. So if you take this leap, be careful. You may not be able to leap back.

The other danger lies in the door itself. You may be able to enter. You may be able to exit. Perhaps you can even exit when and where you wish. But that does not mean you are the only one. There are other beings out there that can do the same. And some of them are purely interdimensional beings that dwell purely in between realms. Watch yourself as you travel along the Stairway between Realms. Protect yourself. But more importantly, protect time and space itself. If you risk releasing one of these beings out into your dimension or another, be responsible. Find another route.

There was once a man named Leonard How lite. He was a dimensional passenger who rode for most of his life on the Stairway between Realms. He fancied himself quite the expert. But Leonard How lite had passed along the Stairway between Realms all of ten to twenty times. He'd seen thirty-five realms, despite only using the passage between them twenty times. Still, for all his knowledge of the passage and the few places he had traveled to, he did not have the sense to take precautions. For example, he never disguised himself or masked his identity. If he traveled to the future or past, he wore his own features like a mask.

He thought that if he was not in his own dimension, there was no fear.

Wrong! Leonard How lite met many versions of himself on his trip through the Stairway between Realms? And upon meeting himself, he created a paradox in that dimension that sent its native Leonard How lite into a pocket. The pockets would hold that Leonard there until the paradox untangled itself. Of course, this really bummed Leonard How lite out. He had gone back at one point to help himself out. Not possible, it seemed.

Another troublesome situation also burst out of the Stairway between Realms thanks to Leonard How lite. You see, he passed between the dimensions with relative ease, but believed he was all alone in that passage. Of course, he was wrong. The shifters, beings that shift between dimensions, stalked Leonard How lite through the passage and were set loose upon several dimensions. Learning this, Leonard did go back and salvage what he could. Most of those universes were already lost, however.

Now, to be fair to Leonard, he's saved the multiverse several times. On multiple occasions, he's undone someone else's dimensional catastrophe. He's untangled paradox for other folks, slew many shifters, and unjumbled the space-time stream in general. He's also trained many individuals on proper Stairway between Realms protocol. So remember, you can be like Leonard How lite. Or you can be like Leonard How lite. Your choice!

Exercise

What's Your Name?

Exercise time: 10 minutes

Benefits: Fosters expression and increases self-esteem

MATERIALS: Assorted markers, 1 sheet of 18-by-24-inch heavy-weight drawing paper

1. Using block letters, write your name in any color on your paper from left to right.

2. Think of a positive word that has the same first letter as your name. Add this word to your drawing in any location on the paper.

3. Pick your favorite colors and create a design inside the letters of your name

Chapter 45. Lemonade

The anticipation overcomes me and I feel my hot, wet pussy throbbing in the middle of the night. I slip out of my tiny lacey underwear and toss them onto the floor. I slowly move my hand towards my pulsating pussy. I know that I won't take long to orgasm because I'm basically already there. Suddenly, I hear a loud noise coming from my front door. My sexual panting turns into pants of fear. I have no idea what that noise might be and I spring out of bed to find out. I quickly make it to my front window. I get the nerve to peer through my blinds to take a look. The entrance light is off but the moonlight shines brightly on a huge dog. It had run up next to my front door and had broken a ceramic flower pot that my best friend Laurie gave me. That explained the loud noise. I decided to check on the dog. I opened the front door slowly hoping there wouldn't be a weirdo there with the dog. Nobody was there. The dog was alone. I bent over to check the tag dangling from its collar when I suddenly felt a very quick shot of cool air. I jumped out of bed up so quickly when I heard the loud noise that I forgot to slip my panties on. The cool air hitting my bare, smooth, pink pussy felt awesome and got me even hotter. I inspected the dog tag thoroughly and started to memorize the phone number on it when suddenly I was startled by the noise of loud steps. I gasped quickly as I saw a shadow creep up behind me. "I'm so sorry I scared you and I apologize for my dog. I just moved into the neighborhood last week and my dog got out from the backyard. He's been gone all day. I was driving home late from work and he ran right in front of my car so I decided to stop and see where he ran to." I knew this guy had gotten a glimpse of my glistening pussy by the way he looked at me from head to toe and by how he couldn't quite look me in the eye as we spoke. "That's ok! I understand. The loud noise just scared the fuck out of me! I'm Alexa, by the way," I said as I tried to hold my short silk night gown down over my thighs as the cool wind blew. "Hi, I'm Bryce, your new neighbor from down the street." As we shook hands, I noticed some small drops of blood on the front porch. "Oh my God, I think your dog may be hurt. Why don't you come inside and check him out? It's a little chilly out here," I told Bryce. "Are you sure that's ok?" he asked. "Yes, of course," I said as I opened the door, lead them in, and went to look for a first aid kit. As Bryce made his way into my home, I noticed that he was very attractive and very, very muscular and well built. He was wearing a white long sleeve shirt and black slacks. It was obvious that he had not made it home from work yet so I knew his story was true. He rolled up his sleeves and started inspecting his dog as I sat on the loveseat next to him. I was very curious about how he would act knowing that I wasn't wearing any panties. Would he make a comment or just overlook it in a gentlemanly manner? At this point, I was so attracted to this almost-stranger named Bryce that I really wished he would make a comment about my "lack of panties". Then I would have a reason to show him more of me. "How long have you lived here?" he asked. He didn't let me answer and instead added more. "My ex-wife and I had to sell the house to settle our divorce and here I am." Ohhhhhh baby, YES!! He's freshly divorced and needs a good FUCK!! My pussy juices start flowing and I respond quickly. "I'm sorry about your divorce. I'm sure things will be better now." "Well, they are much better now that I have met you.

You are absolutely gorgeous!" "Awww...thanks." I tell him. "Would you like something to drink? I have tea and lemonade. " "I would love some, thank you," he said. I get up from the loveseat and walk to the kitchen. My nightgown is short enough that I know he got a very good look at my ass sticking out from underneath as I walked towards the refrigerator. I turn to catch him looking and giggle. "I'm so sorry. I don't mean to stare but I just can't keep my eyes off you. I think you have a great ass. I'm sure your boyfriend is very proud to have such a beautiful girl." I opened the fridge and bent over to get the carafe of lemonade. "oh, I don't have a boyfriend," I yelled out to make sure he heard me. As I stepped back from the fridge, I felt Bryce right behind me. "I was hoping to hear that because you have made me so fucking hard," he whispered as he grabbed my waist from behind. He started kissing my neck gently as he took the lemonade carafe from my hand and placed it on the granite counter. He stopped and asked, "Do you want me as much as I want you?" I appreciate him for asking. Here was a true gentleman that would love to get to know. I didn't answer his question but instead just pulled him near and started kissing him deeply. He was amazing. His tongue explored my mouth as I started to unbuckle his pants. His big hands moved up and down my back as he turned me back around. He pulled my golden hair aside and started to nibble on the back of my neck. That drove me absolutely crazy! He slipped his hands under my nightgown and cupped my huge DD breasts. He grabbed my hard nipples and started to pinch them gently as I quivered at his every touch. He wasn't wearing any clothes by now and I could feel his full-blown erection as I backed up into it. I moaned at his touch as his hands went on their own adventure. He slipped his hands down to my hot pussy and started to work his magic on my pulsating clit. I was very wet already and wanted him NOW! But Bryce wouldn't have it. He wanted to make love to me not just FUCK me. This told me that he was the loving type...a good guy. He's someone that I would have loved to have met sooner. Not now that I was about to move half-way across the country. Things didn't matter at this moment. I just wanted him inside me as soon as possible! Suddenly, he turned me around and let my nightgown fall to the floor exposing my nude body completely. "I love your body. You look amazing," he told me. A hot feeling overcame every inch of me as I melted in his hands. Bryce lifted me onto the granite counter and I accidentally tipped over the carafe full of ice cold lemonade all over my body. The coldness made my nipples even harder as he started to suck on them and push his face in between my breasts. "Mmmmm, I love your gorgeous breasts. They're so perfect. You're so perfect, Alexa. "I just smiled as he made his way down to my pussy. He opened up my thighs ever so gently and started nibbling his way to my smooth hot spot. Fuck!!! This guy is too good to be true. He knows exactly what to do. He placed his tongue on my hot clit and started to slither his way around my plump pink pussy lips. I was soaking with sweet juices that he absolutely loved to lick. "Mmmmm…baby, you taste like delicious lemonade and I just want to drink you up all night long." Bryce made me moan and groan as he continued to drive me crazy with his tongue. "I want you," I moaned to Bryce. He looked straight into my emerald green eyes, smiled and slipped his huge cock inside me and started to thrust hard. I moaned and groaned at each thrust as he went deeper and harder. He had to have been at least 9 inches long and very thick because he had my tight pussy getting hotter and wetter than ever! "Bryce, fuck me harder. I want to feel all of you inside of me. Drive me hard! Drive me crazy. Come on, baby, fuck me harder," I moaned to him louder and we both came together!

Exercise

FAITH/MEANING

Value: --

Activity: --

Activity: --

Activity: --

Value: --

Activity: --

Activity: --

Activity: --

Chapter 46. Lost City in the Woods

"As I read this and begin to drift comfortably asleep, I don't know whether I will find myself drifting asleep more to the sound of my voice or the words I read or perhaps to the spaces between the words. And as I drift comfortably asleep I'll just read this story to myself."

So, as you listen to me, you can begin to drift comfortably asleep and while you begin to drift comfortably asleep you can allow yourself to get comfortable and allow your eyes to close. And I don't know whether you will drift off to sleep with the words that I use, with the sound of my voice, or perhaps with the spaces between my words.

And you can have a sense of being out bird watching one day. Of being in a little shed, a little bird watching shack, with some binoculars gazing out from this quiet spot.

And you are gazing out through some woodland, over a large valley and you can see different birds in the nearby bits of woodland, but you can also see a large circling bird of prey in the distance in the valley and you can see it so gracefully circling.

Seeming to use almost no effort and you look through binoculars at that graceful bird of prey and you have that unusual experience where, when you watch that through binoculars you shut off from the reality around you and awareness of the shack and awareness of everything else, to almost like you are very near to the bird, almost flying with them.

And while you continue to fly gracefully, you start exploring. And it is as if somehow you have taken over this bird. And a part of you is thinking "Am I still in the shack watching the bird and somehow, I have drifted into a daydream, or was I watching the bird so intensely that I have got into the bird's psyche, somehow managed to get into the bird's mind?". And either way, you go with the experience.

You feel a sense of elegance and grace and you continue exploring. And you are now in an area you have never been before. As a bird watcher you have been and watched birds before. You have even been down and walked through the valley, you have even walked and seen some of that river and the lake, but now you seem to have flown over an area you have never been before. An area of woodland, only you notice something about this woodland.

Your eyesight is so good that you notice subtleties, you notice that some trees are slightly higher up than others and you notice there is a certain pattern to these trees and intuitively something tells you it is worth going down there and investigating.

So you fly down and you are too big to fit through the treetops in this area of the woodland, so you circle around and explore and conclude that you are going to have to land at the beginning of the woodland, but you don't know how well a bird of prey is going to be able to walk from the beginning of the woodland all the way into the woods, but you don't see an alternative, so you fly around and land at the beginning of the woodland and as you come in to land, you bring your wings back, you open them wide, slowing you right down, catching as much wind as possible, catching as much of that air as possible.

And you put your feet out in front of you and you have an odd experience, that just as your feet touch the ground, you become yourself again and you find yourself stood before the woodland.

You are still trying to work out whether this is a dream and whether you have somehow gazed at that bird so intensely that you are now dreaming and having this experience and yet it feels very real and undream-like.

And you think, if it was just a dream wouldn't you just wake up by just deciding this is a dream and deciding to just wake up and yet it doesn't seem like a dream or something you can wake up from. It's not something that bothers you, it is just a curiosity.

You walk into the woods, listening to the footsteps, listening to the different sounds in the woods, noticing how the light changes as you walk into the woods. And the woods are quite dense and you have to push through and work your way through.

And as you push and work your way through the woods, you notice that there are some areas that seem to be a bit higher, areas that seem to be a bit lower, like the woods have built on top of something. But you don't know what and you keep pushing and pushing, until eventually there is an area that is a little bit clearer and you notice that the woods have overgrown over some kind of old building. And as you walk around and explore, you find that it seems to have grown over lots of old buildings.

You keep walking and keep exploring and all you keep finding is more and more buildings like this is a huge area of many buildings. Then you find a bit that looks like a normal bit of land, perhaps a normal outcrop of rock and you decide to go and explore it and you scratch through the plants that have covered it over and you notice that it is a wall of a building that has partially collapsed.

And you follow this wall to see where it leads. It seems like you have found some kind of building that would have been near the centre of this lost city. Then as you keep exploring, you notice an indentation in the ground and you notice that this is where an entrance must have once been. So, you start clearing this entrance space and you find that just behind a bit of rubble is a tunnel heading downwards with some steps.

You walk in to the tunnel and as you do, somehow, oddly, your eyes adapt to be able to see in this tunnel, like somehow you have got some of the abilities of the wild animals in this area. You don't try to understand it because you are too busy thinking that it benefits what you want to achieve, you want to explore this area. So, you head down deeper into this building.

And quite a way down you find a stone slab that you think is probably in front of an entrance to something. And you start pushing around on the stone slab and around on the wall around the stone slab and then somehow, you just take a step and the slab moves aside. And it grinds and moves aside, as you walk through and you find yourself in a vast chamber.

You read the scroll with fascination, with wonder, only vaguely aware of the impact it is going to have positively on you. And you read that this one also includes instructions saying that all the scrolls can be read when held on this pedestal by this golden clasp.

So, you go and get another scroll, you place that on the pedestal and clasp it into place and you watch as the writing transforms, almost like mist and movement and changing of the text, to become readable. And you read that one and it is full of knowledge you never would have known, ancient knowledge, ancient wisdom. Then you get another scroll, putting that one back and notice that that scroll also contains ancient wisdom. And you wonder how long it would take to work your way through the thousands of scrolls full of ancient wisdom in this place.

And you read another scroll and another scroll. Taking in and learning more ancient wisdom. Learning on an instinctive level. Learning that with a certain focus, you can become the animals, you can join the spirit of the animals and somehow you had stumbled across that focus and by stumbling across that focus, allowed you to stumble across this knowledge.

And you read and learn and find this knowledge fascinating. And you realise it would take too long to learn all of this knowledge right now, you decide to continue exploring.

And so, you put the original scroll back in place on the pedestal and make sure all the other scrolls are put away in their places and you explore deeper and deeper into this space.

And as you explore, so you discover a giant underground lake and on that lake is a boat and this lake is totally still and you feel it is so still that it is almost unnaturally still, but then, there is no breeze down here.

Then you see a puzzle on the wall and you know there is no further to go in this chamber, but you think it is curious having a puzzle, so you try and solve the puzzle. And after a while moving things around, trying to work the puzzle out, suddenly you get the puzzle, something inside you clicks and makes it make sense to you and then a secret door opens.

You go through the secret door, going deeper and deeper into this building. And you see a room so large that you can't see the other side of it. You can't see the side on the left or the side on the right, you don't know how the ceiling is being held up in a room this large.

And you walk into the room and after a very, very long time of walking in a straight line so that you don't get lost, just following the markings on the ground, you find yourself at another pedestal, only on this pedestal is a bit confusing, you see a perfectly polished black pebble.

You continue to find your way out and then find your way into the woods. Then you work your way through the wood, back the way you came and when you exit the woods, you don't know how far it is to get back to where you came from.

Exercise

You then allow for an evidence-based conclusion on whether that particular thought is valid or not. Let's say you have this particular belief: "My colleague doesn't like me." You would list down all the possible evidence for this thought, such as "He didn't turn around when I called out his name yesterday," or "He didn't reply to my text message." You then compare these thoughts to evidence like, "He invited me to have coffee during break," and "He offered to drive me to the bus stop because it was raining hard."

You don't stop there but come up with other balanced thoughts, such as, "My colleague is busy just like me and has a lot of other things in his mind, too." Using this technique lets you apply logic to get rid of unreasonable negative thoughts and replace those thoughts with ones that are more balanced and rational

Chapter 47. Grape Harvest

I am taking you to a faraway village in Italy. Here my uncle has a vineyard. My uncle's youngest brother, Raphael, helps with the harvesting. It was raining went I went to visit him last November. I welcome you to the vineyard with my uncle and me.
Lie down in your bed. Relax your shoulders and close your eyes. Allow your arms and legs to stretch and become completely relaxed. You feel total tranquility. Visualize the night sky filled with stars on the ceiling above you. Imagine that your head is laying on a pillow of fragrant and soft rose petals. Imagine that there are candles all around you giving off a soft glow. You are becoming more and more relaxed. You are now at the vineyard with me.
I see the dirt road and dusty road that leads to the harvesting area of the vineyards. I had reached in the evening after a long day of travel because his house is quite a way from the city and his vineyard is outside of the village limits. I stayed at the vineyard for several days in the small guesthouse that is there. That first night I simply ate dinner and fell into a deep sleep, exhausted from all my travel. The vineyard has

a distinctly sweet aroma from the ripening fruit on the vines. There is also a rich and earthy smell from the rich soil. It's almost as if breathing in the air you are once again a child rolling around in the dirt as you play and absorbing some of its essence.

I love nature. I find it magical. However, harvesting grapes and making wine are equally interesting to me. It is quite obvious to all who know me that I am crazy about delicious and juicy grapes. Each and every bite of their flesh gives me a deeper appreciation of the complexity of their flavors and fragrances. To grow good grapes, you need several things: time for the grapes to mature and ripen, knowledge of the different types of seeds and plants, and the correct weather conditions. You also must have the appropriate places to make and store your wines as they ferment.

The growing of grapes takes time. The fruit must be used within hours of harvest or it can be frozen... It can be stored and kept fresh if it is stored correctly. But grapes are not like bananas or apples where you can harvest them before they are ripe and allow them to ripen during the shipping and sale process. Grapes can only ripen while they are still on the vine. Grapes are delicate and require great care and patience when growing them.

There are many common fruits that I can give you examples that can be stored for longer periods of time and are more resilient to the packaging and shipping processes. For example, my uncle and I once spent an hour discussing the viability and packability of citrus fruit. We can store grapefruits, lemons, oranges, even avocados for months without losing quality in the fruit. You can even allow them to stay on their trees for several months without any problems. Grapes are not this way. They require constant care and attention from the time of planting, through the harvesting and into the storage of them. This makes the overhead cost for growing grapes to be much higher than that of the other fruits.

I want to take a break here. I want you to imagine that your lover is closing your eyes with their fingertips. Your eyelashes are brushing the skin just under your eyes. You are falling deeper and deeper into a state of complete tranquility. You are completely relaxed, laying in the grass under a tree.

My uncle also grows exotic lemons, oranges, some apples, and a few other fruits. My uncle loves fruit. Here are some interesting facts that he shared with me. These fruits drop off of their trees when they are completely ripe. If they drop before they have ripened it is called a pre-harvest drop. Farmers stop this from happening by spraying the trees with a chemical spray that is designed specifically to help fruit trees regulate the growth and maturation of their fruit. This process normally takes four to six weeks after the tree blooms. I love eating fully ripened fruit right at the vineyard. There are many advantages to eating locally grown fruits. You can get fruit that has not been sprayed with chemicals and is all-natural. The natural growth without chemical interference not only reduced pollution but it allows the fruit to develop all of its nutrients and flavors. I once picked an apple at my uncle's farm, simply put it under cold water to rinse it off and bit straight into it. It was the tastiest apple I have ever eaten. It was as if a harvest festival happened inside of my mouth.

The fruit that I buy from the market near my home in Bulgaria, Germany just cannot compete with the fresh fruit from my uncle's vineyard and farm. That bite of the apple brought back all those summers that my brothers and sisters and I spent at my uncle's vineyard in Italy. We ate farm-fresh fruit all summer. It was an amazing treat.

As I finished my apple, I saw my uncle off in the distance harvesting berries by hand as he always has done since he was a young man. My entire life, I have always looked forward to my yearly visits to help on my uncle's vineyard and fruit farm.

Take a moment to imagine an apple falling into a pile of hay and sinking down into the hay. The fruit falling and sinking into the hay is like your falling deeper and deeper into relaxation and sleep. This is a natural process. You don't have to do anything, just like the apple didn't have to do anything to fall off a tree and into a pile of hay. You just must allow the natural processes of your body to function as they are designed to function.

Now place your hands on your stomach. As you are becoming more and more relaxed the calmness is spreading through your stomach and abdomen. The muscles from the top of your body to the bottom half of your body are completely relaxed. You are in deep relaxation. Your arms and your legs are completely relaxed. Your neck and back muscles are relaxed. You are laying on your back and feeling total peace and relaxation.

I will sometimes watch the tree shakers that are attached to trees with belts. This is an old-fashioned labor-saving device that still works. We don't need the artificial intelligence machines that we often see being used to harvest fruit now. The traditional still work great.

Our family prefers the traditional methods of growing and harvesting. It is best for the fruit. The fruit is less likely to be damaged when picked by loving human hands. Because we harvest in this way, we get better prices from suppliers and store managers because our fruit is always rated at a higher quality than the fruit from the large, machine run farms.

The process by which fruit ripens is called the senescence. When the tree reaches maturity the fleshy part of the ovary of the flower becomes the fruit. The cells multiply through the process of pollination or the phases of fertilization. This stimulates the raped growth and ripening of the fruit for us. I find the science of harvesting fruit fascinating. This cycle happens differently for different fruits. For instance, lemons mature very differently from apples. The formation of cells in the fruits is identified by protoplasm with which the cells are filled. Plant hormones expand the young cells to grow it from embryonic seeds to have a bigger size and weight. Just like all living things, the reproductive system of the plant is how fruit is created. In fruit, little areas called vacuolated make cavities. These cavities create the food we know as fruit.

It is amazing to think about how diverse fruits are in their make-up, not just their appearance. I am so intrigued by the science of fruit.

Fruits also contain different types of nutrition. For instance, dates, bananas, and apples are high in carbohydrates. Whereas olives and avocados are composed of fatty acids that heal and enrich our bodies and minds. Citric acid is found in citrus fruits like pineapples and lemons. It is why they are called citrus fruits. They are very high in nutrition and vitamin C.

However, fruit does not provide us with proteins. We do however receive malic acid from pears and apples and tartaric acid from grapes.

Many fruits are green as they mature. You see this in a lot of tropical fruits like guavas and bananas. Some fruits are ripe when they are green like some varieties of grapes and apples. These beautiful color changes and varieties are one of the things that make fruit interesting as well as delicious. The moment you take a bite out of your favorite fruit, it melts in your mouth and then disappears into your digestive system through your esophagus. You are refreshed and thankful for its nutrition and flavor as the taste lingers on your tongue and the smell in your nostrils.

Fruits are beautiful. Their cell walls contain chlorophyll which lessens over time as they ripen. As the green pigmentation fades away, it is replaced with carotenoids that give yellow and orange fruits their color and anthocyanins that give the red color to berries and mangoes. These replace the green state as the chlorophyll disappears. Usually, acidic fruits lose their acidity and increase in sweetness due to the high sugar content of this stage as well. That sugar content is the real reason that you love fruit. Our bodies are programmed to love sweet things.

Fruits are perishable. The frequent changes to the physical state of the fruit show how quickly that fruit can perish. You can freeze it to keep for a little longer. However, freezing will make it less flavorful and take away its fruity aroma.

Exercise

Sometimes it's difficult to know when to express your emotions to others, but you can learn to meet your needs without overwhelming your family, coworkers, or friends. Having healthy boundaries means knowing where your limits are. For example, you might not want to divulge your personal life to a coworker or a new friend. It's important to step back and look at your needs in every relationship. What do your boundary walls look like?

BENEFITS:

Develops coping skills and emotional regulation

Prep time:

30 minutes

Exercise time:

30 minutes

MATERIALS:

Assorted markers

1 sheet of 18-by-24-inch heavy-weight drawing paper

Assorted printed paper (newspapers, wrapping paper, designed paper)

Scissors

Glue

STEPS:

1. Take 30 minutes to identify the limits on where you feel comfortable with the people in your life on physical, emotional, and spiritual levels.

2. Give yourself permission to say no.

3. With the markers, draw yourself in the middle of the paper.

4. Glue the assorted papers around your portrait to create a healthy boundary wall.

5. Identify one person you need to establish boundaries for, and draw them outside your healthy boundaries wall.

Chapter 48. Ambien

The rhythmic sounds of dripping water greeted me as I stopped just inside the entrance to the cave as the sun sank below the horizon. I forced my inhales to match the slow drip. Only after I'd calmed myself, did I stride forward.

Zagan, one of my mares, saluted. "My liege."

I returned his gesture then continued past. My objective lay in the heart of this cave. I took a hard right and ducked to avoid the low archway.

"Report."

Morfran, one of my commanders, bowed low before me. "It wasn't easy finding her, my liege. They tried to hide her, moving her between palaces. It took patience, but we finally secured her when she emerged from your sons' residence."

No surprise. They'd done the same trying to hide Alissandra. I met Velma's gaze. Even in the dim light of the cave, it was easy to see her wings tucked tightly, but she'd thrown back her shoulders. Clenched fists rested on her hips as she tried to stare me down. There was no repentance, let alone fear in her. Silly child.

"Good work, Morfran. Dismissed." I nodded at Bate, the other guard, to leave us as well. This was a family matter that demanded discretion.

Alfreda sat rigid on the moss-covered bed, face drawn. My men had followed orders, that much was clear judging by the dark circles under her eyes. The bruise on her cheek disturbed me though. What measures had they been forced to go to to withhold sleep? And did she bear any other marks? I pushed the thought away. I'd address her treachery after.

I refocused on my eldest. "Your sister told me you were the one who facilitated Alissandra's... exodus to Wake."

"Escape, you mean?" Velma corrected.

Was she trying to infuriate me? Surely, she didn't expect me to dismiss her behavior and let it go unpunished, but to anger me further was unwise, even for her.

"Semantics. So you admit it?" I continued.

"It was the best option in my judgment," Velma replied.

Matter of fact. No cowering despite what she surely had to know would happen. I respected that.

Alfreda whimpered behind her. "I didn't want to, Velma. He forced it out of me."

Her cowering tone got under my skin, and I couldn't crush a growl. She'd been so strong under my questioning. Now she just sounded pitiful.

Velma didn't break eye contact with me. "I'm sure he did, sister. I hold no ill will against you. No doubt you held out as long as you could."

"I must say I am impressed that you discovered a way to send your sister. It's not common knowledge that it's possible. There have been a few others who have made the journey, but never in such a fashion."

Velma tried to hide her surprise at what I revealed, but her eyes grew large before she could school her expression again. Alfreda sucked in a breath and drew a hand to her mouth.

"Why are you telling me this, Father?" Velma asked.

"Can't I praise my daughter?"

She didn't speak or break her stare.

"By doing what you did, I'm sure you realize you've created a problem for me. Yes, others of the gods have heard about it. Temis, Thena, they're just the ones I know of, but I'm sure there will be more."

Velma's expression didn't change, but Alfreda's eyes grew large. At least one of them was sharp enough to understand. Yes, Alfreda's look told me she remembered my reaction when the regents I'd appointed to oversee the provinces challenged my authority and forced us all into a war—several goaded me over it for eons, calling me weak. I'd vowed never to allow it to happen again. Why oh why did it have to be my own daughter who'd challenged me?

"I am your Father, but perhaps you've forgotten I am also your sovereign. Velma, you have been disloyal, treasonous even. Do you know what the punishment for treason is?"

Velma clenched her jaw but made no reply.

How I respected her. If only every member of my family were as strong.

"Before I pronounce sentence, I want you to understand the full depth of what you did in convincing your sister to become mortal, because I'm not sure you do. If you did, I doubt you would have encouraged her." I took a deep breath. "Velma, to be mortal is to become less. You've sentenced your sister to death, but worse, you've condemned her to grieve the passing of those she loves."

Velma shifted her wings.

Yes, she should be uncomfortable. I continued, pressing my point. She needed to understand. "As gods, the only time we are touched by tragedy is when we care for a mortal beyond helping them dream.

When we become attached, we expend our energies doing what we must to care for them. It's our own choice to make, but if we do, it means we are no longer free. And worse than being a parent caring for the welfare of our immortal children, we are brought low and suffer because of their frailty. I should not have to remind you of Dyeus's grief and lamenting over his son Sarpedon's death. Or Thetis's knowledge that her son Chilles's life would be short and full of grief. She was reduced to groveling and making bargains with others of us gods in desperate attempts to save him. It was hard to watch. What she endured, I would not wish upon anyone, despite her bringing it on herself. She was shortsighted."

Velma shifted her wings again. "With all due respect, Father, I believe that loving has made Ali stronger and more courageous. Before her current charge, she was naïve and easily swayed. But as she has come to understand how she truly, deeply feels about him, she has taken a stand and will defend him, no matter what. She's grown in ways I never would have imagined. Yes, she will necessarily endure grief, but she can live fully, completely. Mortals, through their very mortality, have the potential for great nobility. Our lives seem trivial in comparison."

"You speak so highly of their lesser state, daughter. Do you wish me to send you to Wake? To make you human? Is that what you're saying?"

Velma's gaze held for several heartbeats before she looked away.

"I thought as much. Yours are the ideals of a spoiled child who has never experienced any degree of adversity."

Alfreda shot up, wings flaring. "Velma is not a spoiled child! No doubt she feels she needs to stay to protect us. You act like all you sought was Ali's good. You tortured her just like you're torturing me!"

"That's enough, Alfreda. I will deal with you shortly. Trust me when I tell you, you do not want me addressing your conduct until your sister and I have resolved this issue. Sit down and wait your turn quietly."

Alfreda glared for several heartbeats but at length she furled her wings once more and reseated herself on the mattress.

"That's a good girl. At least one of you obeys."

I returned my focus to Velma. "So now that you understand my perspective, perhaps you can understand the error of your ways."

Velma clenched her jaw. "We shall have to agree to disagree, Father."

I nodded. "I see. Very well, then I shall have to effect a punishment that may assist you in reaching my conclusion."

Alfreda sucked in a breath. I ignored her.

"As your sovereign, I would be well within my rights to have you executed for treason."

I watched for Velma to react. She did not. She must have steeled herself for this outcome. My pride in how I'd raised her grew.

"But as your father, that would cause me to grieve, exactly what I wish to avoid for it would make me appear even weaker. So, I believe I have a fitting punishment that will also help instruct." I turned toward the archway. "Morfran!" My bellow echoed through the cave.

"Yes, my liege." My soldier strode forward and bowed low.

"Have Zagan and Bate join us as well."

Alfreda tensed visibly. I doubted she could gather her wings any tighter. Velma's eyes darted between me and the three guards as they appeared.

"Velma, it is up to you how you endure your punishment. You may do it with dignity or without, but my men will ensure it is carried out."

I turned to Morfran. "Cleave her wings."

"No! You're a beast!" Alfreda shouted, rising. "Velma!"

I nodded for Bate to restrain Alfreda, which he did, despite her kicking and flapping.

She was trying my patience. I boomed, "Alfreda, if you cannot control yourself, you will force me to have him shackle you."

"Sister, don't resist for my sake. He's already hurt you enough. He can do whatever he wants to my body, but he will never break me. Never again," Velma ground out. Alfreda stilled, but tears flowed freely down her cheeks.

With order again restored, I nodded to Morfran.

"Kneel," he commanded. Then turning to the other guard, he said, "Zagan, hold her down."

Velma complied without coaxing, kneeling three strides from me. She would take her punishment with dignity. Wise. I expected nothing less.

Zagan forced her forehead to the ground, fully exposing her wings. She didn't even try to tuck them. Alfreda whimpered but didn't fight Bate.

Morfran removed his sword from its sheath. "Extend your wings fully or I won't be responsible for cutting your back too."

Velma's wings trembled as she stretched them wide, their full span. The shaking grew the longer she held them open. They weren't the largest among my children, but they were certainly noteworthy. I just hoped she learned the lesson I hoped to teach her through this, that becoming less would never make her noble. That notion needed to stop before she led more of my children astray.

I watched her. I didn't need to see her face to know she hadn't yet learned the lesson. The vein bulging in her neck told me as much.

Morfran held the blade up and, with one swift motion, brought it down and across the stem of one wing.

Exercise

What's Your Name?

Exercise time: 10 minutes

Benefits: Fosters expression and increases self-esteem

MATERIALS: Assorted markers, 1 sheet of 18-by-24-inch heavy-weight drawing paper

1. Using block letters, write your name in any color on your paper from left to right.

2. Think of a positive word that has the same first letter as your name. Add this word to your drawing in any location on the paper.

3. Pick your favorite colors and create a design inside the letters of your name

Conclusion

These tales are relaxing to hear, and perfect for those who need to catch some Zest. With each story, you were whisked away into a far-off place, a dream land where people, places, and things aren't as they seem. Where everything seems almost...surreal in a sense. Understanding that is of course, a great way to understand these stories, putting them all together so that you can hear a great tale, and one that's deep, but also relaxing as well.

With that being said, I hope these ten tales will help with sleeping. They are whimsical pieces, and they are quite fun. You've heard the many adventures that either put you in the place of the main character, or you heard some fun, interesting stories that you won't want to ever forget. These unforgettable tales will help lure anyone to sleep, no matter how good, or how bad their sleep schedule is.

Just listen to one of every night before you go to bed, and you'll go straight to dream and, whisked off by the adventures you hear through the words uttered.

So, there you have it, I hope you're able to get yourself some sleep that's worthwhile and filling.

There are many ways that these stories can be used. I gave a lot of thought to the best way to present them, whether to present them to be read at bedtime, or as you would find them if you listened to them so that you can record them in your own voice and at a pace that is comfortable for yourself or perhaps for someone else to listen to. For other hypnotherapists, they can be used like scripts in therapy sessions to help clients to tackle anxiety, worry and stress.

The main reason for writing these stories down was for my Dan Jones Hypnosis YouTube channel subscribers. I have often been asked by my subscribers whether I would release of my stories. It is common to get messages from people saying that they never make it to the end of any of the stories, they are always asleep long before the end and they would love to read the stories to know how they go and how they end. With this in mind, I decided that the best way to present these stories is as authentic as possible to how they are on YouTube.

If you decided to read these stories to help you sleep at night I recommend that you read them in a specific way. It is no good reading through a story fast, in an upbeat voice, or skim-reading. The two ways to read are either to read the stories exactly as they are written and where it talks about "listening to me" or "listening to my voice" you can interpret this to mean that inner voice you are using, as if you are listening to your inner voice talking to you. Alternatively, you can change these words and phrases to suit what you are doing, so that they match your ongoing experience. For example, instead of saying "as you listen to me and begin to drift comfortably asleep, I don't know whether you will find yourself drifting asleep more to the sound of my voice or the words I use, or perhaps to the spaces between my words. And as you drift comfortably asleep I'll just tell a story in the background."

As you read a story, you want to read slowly in a calm and relaxed voice, whether you do this in your head or out loud. You want to have plenty of pauses at times which feel comfortable and natural for you, often at full stops and shorter pauses at commas. Add additional calming emphasis when reading relaxing words and phrases like "begin to relax" and "deeper."

I hope you have pleasant dreams, and I hope you're able to sleep soundly.

Made in the USA
Monee, IL
14 December 2022